Telephone Medicine
Triage and Training
for Primary Care

D0321951

SECOND EDITION

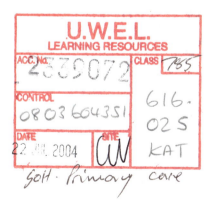

Telephone Medicine

Triage and Training for Primary Care

Harvey P. Katz, MD

Associate Clinical Professor of Pediatrics
Department of Ambulatory Care and Prevention
Harvard Medical School
Harvard Pilgrim Health Care
Boston, Massachusetts

F. A. DAVIS COMPANY • Philadelphia

F. A. Davis Company
1915 Arch Street
Philadelphia, PA 19103

Printed in the United States of America

Last digit indicates print number: 10 9 8 7 6 5 4 3 2

Acquisitions Editor: Margaret M. Biblis
Developmental Editor: Bernice M. Wissler
Cover Designer: Louis J. Forgione

As new scientific information becomes available through basic and clinical research, recommended treatments and drug therapies undergo changes. The authors and publisher have done everything possible to make this book accurate, up to date, and in accord with accepted standards at the time of publication. The authors, editors, and publisher are not responsible for errors or omissions or for consequences from application of the book, and make no warranty, expressed or implied, in regard to the contents of the book. Any practice described in this book should be applied by the reader in accordance with professional standards of care used in regard to the unique circumstances that may apply in each situation. The reader is advised always to check product information (package inserts) for changes and new information regarding dose and contraindications before administering any drug. Caution is especially urged when using new or infrequently ordered drugs.

Library of Congress Cataloging-in-Publication Data

Foreword

In Chapter 1 of this remarkable volume, Dr. Harvey Katz makes the case in numerical terms for the importance of "telephone medicine," observing that telephone calls account for an impressive percentage of all patient contacts in pediatrics (28.5%), internal medicine (24.6%), obstetrics and gynecology (19.6%), and family practice (19.4%). My good wife, Nancy, stated the case in a different way when our son and only child was about 3 years old. Following the advice of the Childbirth Education Association instructors, even before his birth we had sought recommendations for a pediatrician and visited that physician's office to have a "get acquainted" interview. In the subsequent 3 years, many of our most pressing questions and needs for advice "from the pediatrician" had been met, and quite successfully, by advice from the office nurse practitioner over the telephone. "Had I known then what I know now," Nancy said, "we would have had our get acquainted visit with the nurse practitioner and arranged to conduct the visit by telephone!"

Whatever the perspective from which one sees the issue, clinical consultation by telephone for the purposes of symptom interpretation, reassurance, advice on whether or when to come for further clinical evaluation, and self-care is an important element of practice today. Dr. Katz also makes another simple but telling observation. In many respects, telephone practice is the "front door" for most primary care practices. The larger population who looks to us for care, although they may be relatively well most of the time, forms an impression of our interpersonal skills, receptivity, and capacity for support of them in their times of illness on the basis of contacts that are telephone-based. If we act uncourteously or are inattentive to their needs for sound advice by telephone, we will lose the confidence and trust of our patients and their families even before we meet them face-to-face.

The mix of chapters in this user-friendly volume is just what we need to improve on our performance in the sector of telephone medicine. The chapters emphasize the need for a systems approach to a telephone-based practice, help us understand the medicolegal risks entailed in advice-at-a-distance, place major emphasis on the interpersonal aspects ("the art") of telephone-based interaction, provide resources for training and evaluating staff involved in telephone-based communication, and outline useful approaches to providing advice for the kinds of common symptoms that account for the largest proportion of all patient complaints brought to primary care practices. Each of the symptom-focused chapters is evidence-based, highlights the critical elements of information that may be obtained by telephone interview, and makes thoughtful suggestions for follow-up, including suggestions for the timing of in-person visits when needed. All of these chapters are worth reading thoughtfully once, and many will serve as handy resources at the desk when telephone encounters are actually occurring.

This book will grow in importance with time. We all lead increasingly busy lives and need information in a time-critical fashion. This assertion is as true for patients as it is for clinicians. Telephone-based medicine will be part of our technologic approach to alleviating this time crunch and *Telephone Medicine* is an excellent guide to successful use of this technology.

Harvey Katz is precisely the person who should put this volume together. His experience in two major health maintenance organizations, substantial record as an educator in primary care, and contributions to health services research prepare him optimally for the task. In the second edition of *Telephone Medicine*, he has continued to write the pediatric chapters himself while pulling together an able team of practitioners and educators to write the guides for telephone triage of symptoms in adults.

Thomas S. Inui, ScM, MD
Paul C. Cabot Professor and Chairman
Department of Ambulatory Care and Prevention
Harvard Medical School
Harvard Pilgrim Health Care
Boston, Massachusetts

Preface

Even as electronically linked communication such as e-mail and the Internet moves into health care, the telephone continues to ring loud, clear, and non-stop in virtually every medical office and health care facility. In the first edition of this book (1982) and its 1990 revision, I wrote, "One of the strongest links in the chain of communication between patient and physician is the telephone" and "Managing the telephone represents one of the great challenges of ambulatory medical practice." Both of these statements still ring true, perhaps even more so. The volume and complexity of calls to medical practices today is astronomical, and the telephone is a leading cause of patient complaints and staff burnout from job stress. Volume overload, deficient systems, lagging use of technological advances, and suboptimal training of staff account for many of these problems.

Unlike its predecessors, this edition addresses the telephone care needs of both the pediatric and adult populations. It is written for triage nurses, nurse practitioners, physician assistants, medical students, pediatricians, family physicians, internists, and house staff. In addition, medical assistants and other support staff, as integral members of the health care team, should also find this material useful in performing their highly important jobs.

As implied by the title, *Telephone Medicine: Triage and Training for Primary Care*, the foundation needed to improve telephone care comprises an interconnected triad of **telephone medicine** (systems and technology), **triage** (protocols and communication skills), and **training** (staff preparation and quality improvement). That is the emphasis of the book. We touch on the promise and problems in the use of e-mail and recent developments in telephone-linked care, but speculation about the role of emerging advances in communication technology is beyond the scope of this book.

The core objectives of this edition remain:

- To provide practical, useful, and accessible information to practicing clinicians and their staff
- To provide time-tested protocols for responding to the calls most commonly received in primary care practice, both pediatric and adult
- To help triage staff make timely decisions that safely minimize inappropriate utilization of office visits and emergency services
- To serve as both a reference book and a resource for training and self-study
- To guide patients in using the telephone more effectively

To achieve those objectives, we have included features such as:

- The requirements for high-quality in-office call centers and after-hours programs

- Recommendations for implementing office software to monitor key telephone care parameters, such as time on hold and abandonment rate, and for using these measurements to improve telephone service

- Lessons to be learned from real malpractice cases in which telephone triage in the office was the basis of the claim
- Guidelines for prescribing medication over the telephone
- Triage protocols (Telephone Decision Guidelines) written by highly experienced primary care clinicians, providing clear and specific guidance as to whether appointments are indicated, and how urgently
- Clustering of high-priority protocol questions to expedite the determination of whether emergency services are needed
- Sound home management advice for adults and children not in need of an office visit
- Highlighting of key information for immediate recognition and reference
- A universally applicable four-step approach to staff training, including examples of audit forms to use in role-playing or monitoring
- Practical advice for staff on the art of satisfying patients on the telephone and creating a positive image for the practice

The triage staff are specialists who have an exquisitely vital but difficult job. It is my hope that this new edition will alleviate the pressure for the triage staff and the busy practitioner, and will help to improve both the efficiency and quality of care that patients receive when they call.

Harvey P. Katz, MD
Boston, Massachusetts

Acknowledgments and Dedication

I am greatly indebted to a number of people for their inspiration and help in making this second edition of *Telephone Medicine: Triage and Training for Primary Care* a reality:

To my patients and their families, who have allowed me the privilege of caring for them and teaching me more than they know.

To the telephone triage staff with whom I have worked for so many years. They have had great impact on the health care of families and have my admiration and respect for performing this difficult task with great skill.

To my primary care practice teammates—pediatricians, nurses, and support staff. It has been the support and nursing staff who have performed the lion's share of triage responsibilities so ably.

To my specialty colleagues—internists, family physicians, nurse practitioners, and physician assistants—who have combined to create this edition's unique multi-specialty approach to telephone triage.

My special thanks to Bernice Wissler, Senior Developmental Editor at F. A. Davis, whose eagle eye, sharp wit, and red flags have been so invaluable.

Finally, I express gratitude and appreciation to my family, as I dedicate this book to my wife Marion and children Tamara, David, and Tanya, for their understanding and unending support as they acclimated to the constant ring of the telephone in our home.

About the Author

Dr. Katz is an Associate Clinical Professor of Pediatrics at the Harvard Medical School in the Department of Ambulatory Care and Prevention. Dr. Katz completed his pediatric residency at the Johns Hopkins Hospital in Baltimore, Maryland, and received his Doctor of Medicine from the Downstate Medical Center in Brooklyn, New York, following his B.A. degree from Hamilton College in upstate New York.

Following his residency at Hopkins, Dr. Katz served as a Captain in the US Army Medical Corps at Tripler Army Hospital, where he developed a large primary care pediatric practice and a pediatric endocrine consultation service for the military, and also served as senior faculty for the Army's pediatric residency training program. After leaving the Army, Dr. Katz entered fellowship training in pediatric endocrinology at the University of California, San Francisco.

Dr. Katz returned to Johns Hopkins, where he continued his combined interests in patient care, teaching, and research, and became the founding physician of Hopkins' innovative health care delivery system, the Columbia Medical Plan, in Columbia, Maryland. During his 16-year tenure, Dr. Katz was Chief of Pediatrics and Associate Medical Director of the Medical Plan, and an Associate Professor of Pediatrics and Pediatric Endocrine Attending at the Johns Hopkins School of Medicine.

In Columbia, Dr. Katz continued his pediatric practice and was actively involved in the community as a Day Care and Early Childhood Education consultant, a member of the American Academy of Pediatrics Committee on Adoption, and a member of the Howard County Commission for the Handicapped. His long-standing interest in the role of the telephone in patient medical care began in the early 1970s. The first edition of his book was first published in 1982 as the *Telephone Manual of Pediatric Care*. It underwent major revision in 1990, including a change to the present title.

In 1985, Dr. Katz accepted a position as Health Center Medical Director for the Harvard Community Health Plan, and moved to Boston, joining the Harvard faculty. Dr. Katz is active in local and national continuing medical education for physicians and nurses. He is deputy director of Primary Medicine Today, known as Pri-Med, the nationally recognized Harvard continuing medical education conference in primary care medicine. He teaches medical students in their primary care clerkship and lectures nationally on primary care, telephone medicine, and pediatric endocrine topics.

Dr. Katz's wife teaches English as a second language in the public school system. He has three children and one grandchild.

Contributors

William T. Branch, Jr., MD
Carter Smith, Sr. Professor of Medicine
Vice Chair of Primary Care
Director, Division of General Medicine
Emory University School of Medicine
Atlanta, Georgia

William D. Carlson, MD, PhD
Assistant Professor of Medicine
Harvard Medical School
and
Attending Physician
Brigham and Women's Hospital
and
Director of Cardiovascular Research
Harvard Vanguard Medical Associates
Boston, Massachusetts

Phyllis L. Carr, MD
Assistant Professor of Medicine
Harvard Medical School
and
Assistant Visiting Physician
Massachusetts General Hospital
Boston, Massachusetts

Christopher P. Cheney, MD, PhD
Gastroenterology Service
Walter Reed Army Medical Center
Washington, District of Columbia
and
Uniformed Services University of the Health
  Sciences
Bethesda, Maryland

Ina Cushman, PA-C
Senior Physician Assistant, Surgical
  Specialties
Harvard Vanguard Medical Associates
Braintree, Massachusetts

Robert H. Fletcher, MD, MSc
Professor
Department of Ambulatory Care and
  Prevention
Harvard Medical School
Harvard Pilgrim Health Care
Boston, Massachusetts

John D. Goodson, MD
Associate Professor of Medicine
Harvard Medical School
and
Physician
Massachusetts General Hospital
Boston, Massachusetts

David E. Katz, MD
Department of Enteric Infections
Division of Communicable Diseases and
  Immunology
Walter Reed Army Institute of Research
Washington, District of Columbia
and
Assistant Professor of Medicine
Uniformed Services University of the Health
  Sciences
F. Edward Hébert School of Medicine
Bethesda, Maryland

William F. Kelly III, MD
Fellow, Pulmonary and Critical Care Medicine
Walter Reed Army Medical Center
Washington, District of Columbia

Juliet K. Mavromatis, MD
Assistant Professor of Medicine
Emory University
Atlanta, Georgia

William J. Mullally, MD
Clinical Instructor in Neurology
Harvard Medical School
and
Director of the Headache Program
Harvard Vanguard Medical Associates
Braintree, Massachusetts

Marie-Eileen Onieal, MMHS, RN, CPNP
Immediate Past President
American Academy of Nurse Practitioners
Austin, Texas
and
Health Policy Coordinator
Bureau of Health Quality Management
Massachusetts Department of Public Health
Boston, Massachusetts

Martin A. Quan, MD
Professor of Clinical Family Medicine
Family Practice Residency Director
UCLA School of Medicine
Los Angeles, California

Laurence J. Ronan, MD
Deputy Director of Primary Care
Harvard Medical School
and
Director
Harvard Combined Medicine and Pediatrics
    Program
Massachusetts General Hospital
Boston, Massachusetts

Jeannette M. Shorey, MD
Assistant Professor
Department of Ambulatory Care and
    Prevention
Harvard Medical School
Harvard Pilgrim Health Care
Boston, Massachusetts

Jane S. Sillman, MD
Instructor in Medicine
Harvard Medical School
and
Director
Primary Care Residency Program
Brigham and Women's Hospital
Boston, Massachusetts

Susan Stangl, MD, MSEd
Associate Professor
Assistant Dean for Student Affairs
Department of Family Medicine
UCLA School of Medicine
Los Angeles, California

Frank J. Twarog, MD, PhD
Associate Clinical Professor
Harvard Medical School
and
Senior Associate in Medicine
Division of Immunology
Children's Hospital
Boston, Massachusetts

Deborah J. Wald, MD
Assistant Program Director
Harvard Combined Medicine and Pediatrics
    Residency Program
and
Assistant in Medicine and Pediatrics
Massachusetts General Hospital
and
Instructor in Medicine and Pediatrics
Harvard Medical School
Boston, Massachusetts

Richard S. Weinhaus, MD
Eye Health Services
Quincy, Massachusetts

Richard N. Winickoff, MD
Associate Professor of Medicine
Harvard Medical School
and
Medical Director
MGH Beacon Hill Primary Care and
    MGH Downtown
Boston, Massachusetts

Contents

SECTION FOUR
TELEPHONE TRIAGE: SYMPTOMS IN ADULTS

SECTION FIVE
TRAINING AND EVALUATING TELEPHONE STAFF

SECTION ONE

· ·

THE TELEPHONE IN THE PRIMARY HEALTH CARE PRACTICE

Harvey P. Katz, MD

CHAPTER 1

· · · · · · · · · · · · · ·

The Role of the Telephone in Medical Care—An Overview

When Alexander Graham Bell received the first telephone patent in 1876, no one could have dreamed how profoundly the telephone would affect the practice of medicine. The telephone has become the piece of equipment used most often by clinicians worldwide. And now, with cellular phones and other technology, the doctor truly is no farther away than the closest telephone or computer. Managing the ever-increasing volume of calls and demand for telephone access has become a major challenge for all specialties, however. Depending on the field, telephone contacts account for between 11 and 50% of all medical encounters. In primary care, telephone encounters make up 12 to 28% of contacts, of which up to half result in the need for further evaluation. Telephone calls account for 28.5% of all patient contacts in pediatrics, 24.6% in internal medicine, 19.6% in obstetrics and gynecology, and 19.4% in family practice.[1,2]

The phone is a double-edged sword: It is both an invaluable communication link between health care professionals and their patients and a focal point for patient complaints about poor service. In one study of Denver and Baltimore pediatricians, over half of the respondents considered the telephone the most frustrating part of their practice. Problems within telephone medicine fit into several general categories:

- Volume overload with access difficulties, particularly acute when practices are short-staffed
- Incomplete training and preparation of telephone staff in the art and skill of telephone triage

1

- A myriad of problems relating to telephone triage and office supports:
  - Using appropriate protocols
  - Poor documentation of telephone encounters
  - Inadequate office systems to support telephone medicine
  - Inappropriately utilizing the skill mix of office staff

The increasing demand for service by telephone and the unpredictability of telephone calls has long been a challenge in primary care. A busy internal medicine practice of 12 clinicians may receive 1000 calls daily, with 50 to 100 occurring during a peak hour. Because they have no warning of each call's content, staff members who handle the telephone must be especially well trained and well integrated into the office systems.

All too frequently the end point of a telephone encounter is frustration, error, or delay in diagnosis, which can result in medical liability. Because it is impossible for the clinician to speak to every patient who calls, the current trend toward delegation of varying degrees of telephone responsibility was inevitable. But just because someone answers the phone, we cannot assume that the person will automatically know what to do. How well are clinicians and medical support staff prepared for this critical office responsibility? The ambulatory care setting in private medical offices provides an excellent environment for such training, which can include a variety of teaching methods such as role playing, critiquing of live tapes, and video script scenarios of telephone encounters. These can be used as springboards for group discussions of telephone management protocols, such as those in Chapters 8 through 62 of this book.

The importance of educating patients (or the parents of pediatric patients) in all areas of telephone use also cannot be overemphasized. Instructions on how patients can best use the telephone should be explicit, as illustrated in Appendix A.

Among the key elements in a successful telephone medicine system, regardless of specialty, are:

- Specialized training in triage
- Designating specific responsibility to triage staff (usually nurses)
- Using appropriate protocols and telephone decision guidelines
- Systematically documenting all medically relevant calls
- Using medical and nurse supervisors to supervise, review, and evaluate performance

It is important that the telephone responsibility be integrated into the fiber of the medical practice. It is a dynamic role and should be periodically reassessed and modified, striving for the highest quality of performance and service. Collecting data on the number and peak times of calls is helpful in this regard, as is the careful analysis of patient complaints, which may lead to improvements as a result of problem solving.

As complicated as a face-to-face patient visit may be, a telephone encounter is even more complex. There is less time, no body language, and rarely an opportunity for second thoughts once the call is over. To improve a telephone system, we must understand it in terms of multiple processes working together. In the heat of a hectic day, it is easy to lose sight of this multitude of complex factors that influence a single telephone encounter:

- The patient and family
- The nature of the call
- The skill and preparation of the staff
- System characteristics
- Supports for the staff
- Medicolegal precautions

CHAPTER 2

Organizing an (
Telephone Care

The requisites and multiple factors that de
with our patients have been discussed in Ch
factors does not happen by chance. Because
tices has increased dramatically, each offic
and implementing a telephone system as is
key to providing the highest quality of patie
well-defined responsibilities to skilled triage
over the processes. These staff members n
training, and measures in order to achieve th

Monitoring the Telephone Syste

Measures are needed to continuously evalua
standards are needed to improve it. For any
improve it. Measures that have been used
following:

- Total number of calls received
- Number of calls per hour
- Average time to answer
- Peak call hours
- Percentage of all calls answered before g
- Wait time in the queue (time on hold)
- Abandonment rate

Table 2–1 shows a set of such telephone sta
partment from 8 A.M. to 5 P.M. Monday throu

Based on benchmarking, patient surveys
data, the following standards are suggeste

- Abandonment rates no greater than 5%
- Average time to answer less than 30 sec
- 90% of all calls answered before enterin

These standards may be difficult to achie
on specific telephone goals and appropriate
automatically is available from telephone co
requires an answering and queuing machin
human voice to answer the call before the co

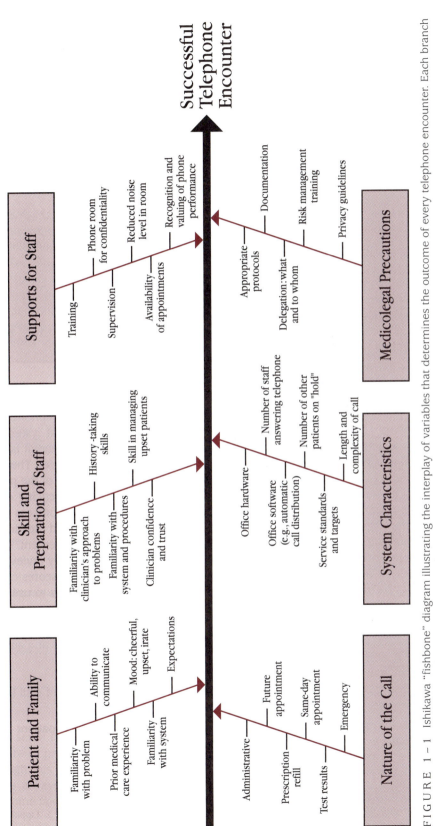

FIGURE 1–1 Ishikawa "fishbone" diagram illustrating the interplay of variables that determines the outcome of every telephone encounter. Each branch represents a process within the total system of telephone medicine.

TABLE 1–1	Telephone Quality-of-Car...

1. Do you know how many phone calls th...
   six reasons for calls?
2. Is the average duration of employment
   greater than 2 years?
3. Has the practice recruited the right per...
4. Does the practice have formalized trair...
   and triage?
5. Does the staff have written protocols, s...
   procedures for routine situations?
6. Does the staff have written protocols fo...
   when physicians or other clinicians are...
7. Does the staff document all medically s...
8. Does the staff write smarter rather thar...
9. Does the staff have a low threshold to b...
10. Has the office been free of patient comp...
    telephone staff in the last month?
11. Do clinicians in the office personally rev...
    regularly with the staff to be sure that o...
    for management by telephone are so m...
12. Have clinicians met with the staff in the...
    telephone and to listen to their problem...

The interplay of all these factors is i...
shown in Figure 1–1. This interplay deter...
counter. Each segment of the diagram rep...
telephone medicine. The *input* is the telep...
response to that request (e.g., an appointm...
sired *outcome* in the successful encounter...
tice is to improve quality and service, les...
tinuous improvement, which starts with th...
makes up the larger system. Small improve...
fication of the root defect in a process lead...
improvement of telephone service in each...
the checklist in Table 1–1. Score one poin...
to 12, congratulations. If it needs improve...
four steps detailed in Chapter 63:

1. Get to know your own system better.
2. Implement a program of study for all...
   (see Chapter 64).
3. Require training of other staff memb...
4. Increase involvement of clinicians in...
   of the staff members who answer the...

The goal of the process should be improve...
staff satisfaction.

REFERENCES

1. Curtis, P: The practice of medicine on the telephone...
2. Katz, HP: Telephone medicine. In Dershowitz, RA...
   Raven, Philadelphia, 1999, p 18.

TABLE 2–1	Telephone Service Statistics						
Day	Total Calls Received	Calls per Hour	Average Time to Answer (Sec)	Peak Hour	% Answered Before Queuing	% Abandoned (of total)	% Answered in 30 Seconds
Monday	409	45	156	9 A.M.	16	23	20
Tuesday	340	38	124	10 A.M.	9	16	31
Wednesday	277	33	48	8 A.M.	30	11	48
Thursday	268	28	56	12 P.M.	45	5.5	56
Friday	205	23	33	1 P.M.	62	4.9	72
Average	300	33	83		30	12	45
Standard			30		90	<5	90

Note: If there are 45 calls per hour (as on Monday) and each telephone assistant can manage 15 calls per hour, 3 people should be the minimum staffing.

the impersonal approach to which many patients and clinicians justifiably have an aversion. In other words, even if there is automated answering, staff members do not have to use it. It can be regarded mainly as a backup as well as a means to record the data for measurements.

> Nothing can replace the human voice. Having a person answer the phone promptly is a practice that should be preserved if possible. For some groups, however, a machine approach has been employed to meet the rising volume of calls.

If the machine approach is chosen, two basic types of instruments can be chosen: Call Processing and Automatic Call Distribution. These usually function together. *Call Processing* is the automatic routing of callers to a desired extension or group of phones. Callers listen to a greeting that describes a number of available options (e.g., emergencies, appointments, pharmacy) and select their choice by pressing a key on their touch-tone phones. When an option is selected from the menu, the call will be routed to the desired location.

Automatic Call Distribution (ACD) distributes telephone calls to departments by queuing callers in the order of their receipt. It consists of hardware and software configured for answering the call and transferring it to staff. When all staff members are busy, the caller hears the all too familiar message that the call will be answered in the order it was received. The waiting time interval may be accompanied by music or a recorded educational message to let callers know they have not been disconnected.

Types of Calls

It is helpful to organize the telephone triage system into incoming calls for problems needing medical assessment versus calls for future scheduled appointments and administrative information. The initial call most frequently is taken by either a medical

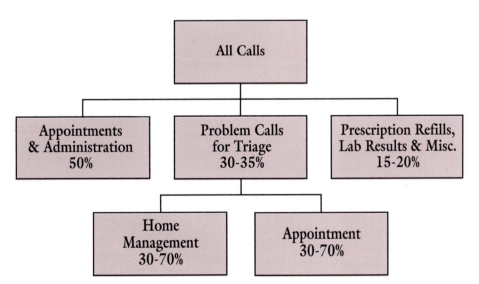

FIGURE 2–1 The calls coming into a clinical practice involve administrative matters as well as illness problems. Depending on the size of the practice, telephone assistants may be assigned responsibility for specific types of calls, but all should be cross-trained so they can handle each type. The disposition of problem calls will vary according to the skill level of the triage specialist and the instructions of the supervising clinician.

TABLE 2-2 **Prioritized Triage Disposition for Common Presenting Complaints**

Emergencies (a suspected life-threatening illness or event)—Activate EMS/911*
A. Airway (compromised or obstructed)
  - Choking
  - Neck or spine injury
  - Croup with cyanosis in any infant or child
B. Breathing problems (severe respiratory compromise)
  - Difficulty breathing from any cause
  - Near drowning
  - Acute allergic (anaphylactic) reaction with respiratory difficulty (food, bee sting, medication)
C. Circulation (suspected or impending shock)
  - Cardiac arrest
  - Any chest pains suggesting possibility of heart attack
  - Uncontrollable bleeding
  - Acute allergic (anaphylactic) reaction (food, bee sting, medication)
  - Poisoning or overdose of medication with change in mental status, signs of shock, or any respiratory difficulty
D. Disability and/or neurologic impairment or paralysis
  - Convulsion (seizure)
  - Any neurologic symptoms suggesting possibility of stroke
  - Coma or unconsciousness
  - Head trauma with behavioral change or any change in mental status
  - Diabetic hypoglycemic reaction with mental confusion and inability to take oral glucose feeding
E. Other
  - Severe trauma (e.g., fall from high place such as tree or building window)
  - Obvious fracture
  - Severe pain and unable to walk
  - Serious suicide attempt or threat
  - Sexual assault

Immediate appointment—As soon as possible (within 2 hours)†
  - Acting very ill (very irritable or lethargic)
  - Severe or increasing abdominal pain or pain localized to the lower abdomen
  - Acute allergic reactions (e.g., hives) without respiratory symptoms or signs of anaphylaxis
  - Extremely anxious parent or acutely depressed patient
  - Burns
  - Sudden change in any condition and symptoms worsening
  - Croup symptoms in infants less than 6 months old
  - Any fever in infants less than 3 months of age
  - High fever (104°F or higher)
  - Head trauma without neurologic symptoms or signs
  - Possible petechial (purplish or blood-spot) rash

Appointment same day or same session—(within 8 hours)‡
  - Diarrhea
  - Earache
  - Fever uncontrolled by treatment
  - Joint pain or swelling
  - Excessive urination and thirst

(Continued)

TABLE 2-2 Prioritized Triage Disposition for Common Presenting Complaints (Continued)

Appointment same day or same session—(within 8 hours)[†]

- Pain or burning on urination
- Skin infection
- Sore throat
- Swollen glands

Future appointment—≤ 3 days or ≥ 4 days[§]

- Recurrent anxiety attacks
- Mild chronic depression
- Diagnostic problems with nonacute symptoms that have been present for a long time (e.g., recurrent headache, chronic abdominal pain)
- Emotional or behavioral problems
- Enuresis (bedwetting) in a child over 4 years of age
- Growth problems
- School problems
- Smoking cessation
- Weight problems

---

*List is not intended to be all-inclusive but rather is a guide for triage. Presenting complaints as outlined may overlap into several A-B-C-D categories. For more detailed qualifiers refer to specific symptom chapters.

[†]These are examples. Judgment is required based on suspected severity, patient or parental anxiety, or potential consequences of condition worsening if not seen immediately.

[‡]These are examples. Judgment is required based on no risk or low risk from not being seen immediately and patient comfort. For detailed triage questions, refer to individual chapters.

[§]Patients are very reluctant to wait, so the appointment should be given as soon as possible, depending on the time available and the nature of the problem. These are examples to serve as guidelines for similar chronic problems.

---

assistant or receptionist, who should be trained in future appointment making and referring calls for problem care to either the triage nurse or the physician. Although the proportions may vary depending on the practice and specialty, generally half of all calls are for future appointments or administrative information (hours, billing, etc.), about one-third are problem calls for triage, and the remainder are requests for prescription refills and laboratory results (Fig. 2–1). Of the problem calls for triage, the percentage that can be managed without an appointment will vary according to the skill and training of the triage staff and the degree to which the supervising clinicians have delegated the responsibility. Therefore the proportion given home management advice may be as low as 30% or as high as 70%, with the remaining callers scheduled to be seen by the clinician or in the emergency room. In a pediatric practice, about 50% of the patients seen by a given clinician are same-day appointments; the comparable number for adult medicine is approximately 25%.

Internists have expressed less confidence in their telephone medicine preparedness than those in other specialties. Although the reasons patients call them are similar to the proportions of types of calls to other primary care practices, the calls internists receive tend to be longer and more complex. Telephone management thus is more variable.[1]

Triage staff should view the timing of appointments in relationship to the presenting complaints (Table 2–2), which can be categorized as:

Life-threatening emergency (activate EMS or 911)
Appointment as soon as possible (within 2 hours)
Appointment during the same session or day (within 8 hours)

Future appointments (within 3 days)
Future appointments (4 days or more)

Administrative Calls and Appointments

Although it may not be feasible to have a separate telephone line for scheduling future appointments, the conceptual separation of future from same-day appointments can be helpful in training and orienting triage staff. As mentioned, more than half of all incoming calls are for either setting up or canceling regularly scheduled appointments or for other administrative purposes such as prescription refills, requests for laboratory results, school and camp forms, and other information about the practice. Staff should be trained to ask all new patients to transfer previous records and to educate patients to call for future appointments after 10:00 A.M. and before 4:00 P.M., to avoid the peak rush of calls reporting illness complaints. Peak hours for calls about illness pertaining to children occur early in the morning and after school. For adults, the peak hours are usually early morning, noon, and early evening. The number of calls increases dramatically on Mondays and after 3-day weekends.

Triaging Problem Calls

About one-third of telephone calls will be for some type of problem care. Triage staff who receive calls about problems must choose between two basic options:

- Provide home management advice
- Schedule an appointment

As mentioned, the skill and training of the triage staff and the clinicians' attitudes will influence the proportion of calls receiving home management advice.

> The most efficient triage systems have the following characteristics:
>
> - RNs as the responsible triage staff members
> - Training program emphasizing problem-care protocols, the art of communication, risk management, and patient confidentiality
> - System of documentation specifically designed for telephone encounters
> - Supervision and evaluation

In one analysis of the frequency distribution for 2520 pediatric telephone encounters, the three most common types of illness complaints reported by telephone were respiratory, gastrointestinal, and dermatologic, which collectively accounted for almost two-thirds of all illness-related complaints. These data can serve as a guide to the content of triage training programs, with a major focus on advice protocols. The percentage of complaints that are managed independently also varies by the nature of the problem; in pediatrics they have been found to range between 22 % of respiratory complaints and 60 % of gastrointestinal complaints (Table 2–3).

Experiences in both fee-for-service[2] and managed care[3] settings have documented high degrees of patient satisfaction with the use of high-quality triage systems in lieu of speaking directly to the clinician. Follow-up of patient calls has confirmed the safety of delegating this responsibility to nurses. Given the increasing demand for telephone management, triage systems not only are more cost effective but also result in higher degrees of clinician satisfaction, allowing clinicians more time to spend with patients who need their attention.

TABLE 2-3 Disposition and Frequency Distribution of Illness Complaints Reported by Telephone to a Pediatric Practice				
Type of Complaint	Number of Calls	Immediate Visit (%)	Advised for Home Care (%)	Referred to Clinician (%)
Respiratory	620	65	22	5
Gastrointestinal	160	27	60	24
Dermatologic	146	39	45	15
Other*	559	42	26	40
Total	1485	43	38	21

*Includes trauma, headache, and symptoms related to the eye, musculoskeletal system, and genitourinary system.

Triaging Emergency Calls

The worst possible scenario for a true emergency is for a patient with a life-threatening condition to be brought into the office rather than being referred directly to an emergency room. For the patient, precious time for prompt emergency treatment is lost; for the primary care practice, the office is totally disrupted and the care of the patients waiting is delayed and rushed. Although the medical management of emergencies is beyond the scope of this book, the telephone management of an emergency situation could not be more relevant. A potential life or death emergency situation can be lurking behind any routine telephone call. Triage staff members must be prepared to manage such calls and make important decisions, even if the clinicians are absent from the office. The recommendation for training in triage of emergency calls is:

- The EMS/911 system should be activated for all life-threatening situations.
- Triage staff should review with the supervising clinician how potential emergency situations that present by telephone should be managed. (See Table 2–2 and Chapters 8 through 62.)
- Whenever there is doubt about a possible emergency situation, the clinician should be interrupted immediately. Protocols and judgment should be used to determine quickly whether an emergency exists.

The more informed triage attendants are regarding questions to ask and procedures to follow, the easier it will be for them to stay calm and mentally alert when an emergency arises.

- The patient's name and phone number should always be obtained early in the conversation if at all possible, in case the call is cut off.
- If a patient is referred to an emergency room, always call the emergency room to give advance notice. If the clinician decides to bring the patient into the office, advance preparations may be needed in terms of both scheduling and equipment.
- A follow-up call should be placed to the emergency room for any patient who is referred there.

Triaging After-Hours Calls (Call Centers)

One recent trend in telephone medicine has been the development of after-hours triage programs (call centers) in both fee-for-service and managed care settings. The growing volume of telephone calls, the need for service to be provided in the most cost-effective way, and the need for clinicians to balance work and home life are the primary drivers for the growth of these call centers. As more clinicians "sign out" evening, night, and weekend calls, the number of such call centers is growing dramatically. (About 30 % of pediatricians now subscribe.) Some call centers are sponsored by hospitals in an effort to increase inpatient and emergency room utilization, some are entrepreneurial, and others have been organized by managed care organizations to meet growing patient demand while also improving the clinicians' work life. Funding may be on a per call, fee-for-service basis; by a subscription fee; or by per member, per month capitation for large managed care organizations.

Some of these programs have been operating for 10 to 15 years and have successfully provided telephone medicine in hundreds of thousands of encounters with no reported major adverse medical or legal outcome and with sustained high levels of patient and clinician satisfaction.

The telephone medicine principles for after-hours call centers and daytime triage are basically the same, with some modifications based on the needs of individual primary care clinicians and groups. Critical elements of successful after-hours programs include:

- Experienced and skilled triage nurses
- Use of established telephone triage protocols and decision guidelines
- Continuous training, evaluation, and supervision
- Close communication and linkage with the primary care clinicians being served, with service and systems tailored to their needs (where and by whom patients should be seen, use of hospitals, sending medical encounter records to the primary care clinician in a timely fashion, such as the morning after a nighttime call)
- Strong medical and nurse leadership and direction

Clinicians interested in subscribing to a call center should carefully evaluate the quality of care, service, and supervision of individual centers before committing the care of their patients. National quality standards are being developed to ensure that these programs meet community standards. A program of accreditation and site visits also is planned.

Other Emerging Trends

Just as Bell's invention of the telephone in 1876 transformed the world of communications, so too is electronically linked communication technology revolutionizing how patients access information and how we "talk" to each other. This intersection of communication and access to information is reshaping the practice of medicine for both patients and health care professionals. Emerging trends in technology, including electronic mail (e-mail), interactive voice response, and telephone-linked care (TLC), influence how patients and clinicians communicate. The specific role of these advances in primary care practice, and other applications of the Internet such as real-time video and telephone calls carried over the Internet,[4] are beyond the scope of this book.

E-Mail

The commonly used Internet service, e-mail, is growing rapidly as a two-way communication substitute for the telephone between patient and clinician. Currently it can be described as a mixture of promise and problems.[5] It is fast, eliminates being put on hold and playing phone tag, is less likely to be overlooked than voice mail, and is instantly self-documented. There are significant privacy and confidentiality issues, however, with a potential for inappropriate and clinically dangerous use and serious medicolegal risk. Further, clinicians could be inundated with so many messages that they would have no time to see patients. Lack of reimbursement for time spent responding to e-mail messages could reduce clinicians' income.

Much depends on the negotiated contract with the patient population and how comfortable clinicians are with the computer in general.[6] There are authoritative guidelines[7] and possible solutions to these potential problems, but it is premature to predict the future impact of this technology on clinical practice and patient-clinician relationships without more experience and research.

Automated Systems

Telephone-Linked Care (TLC) is an automated telecommunication technology in which a human voice is controlled by an Interactive Voice Response (IVR) system. Patients communicate from home using their touch-tone telephone and connect to scripted, branching-question computer-voiced instructions. The application of TLC is now being studied, with promising results, for its impact in improving a variety of health behaviors such as compliance with medication-taking, management of childhood asthma, counseling and relief for caregivers of patients with Alzheimer's disease, screening for mammography, and monitoring of patients with hypertension.[8]

REFERENCES

1. Elnicki, DM, et al: Telephone medicine for internists. JGIM 15:337–343, 2000.
2. Poole, SR, et al: After-hours telephone coverage: The application of an area-wide telephone triage and advice system for pediatric practices. Pediatrics 92:670–679, 1993.
3. Pert, JC, et al: A 10-year experience in pediatric after-hours telecommunications. Current Opinion in Pediatrics. 8:181–187, 1996.
4. Glowniak, J: History, structure, and function of the Internet. Semin Nucl Med 28:135–144, 1998.
5. Mandl, KD, et al: Electronic patient-physician communication: Problems and promise. Ann Intern Med 129:495–500, 1998.
6. Bergeron, BP: Get in with the e-crowd. Digital Doc 107:31–34, 2000.
7. Kane, B, and Sands, DZ, for the AMIA Internet Working Group, Task Force on Guidelines for the Use of Clinic-Patient Electronic Mail: Guidelines for the clinical use of electronic mail with patients. JAMIA 5:104–111, 1998.
8. Friedman, RH: Automated telephone conversations to assess health behavior and deliver behavioral interventions. J of Medical Systems 22:95–101, 1998.

CHAPTER 3

■ ■ ■ ■ ■ ■ ■ ■ ■ ■ ■ ■ ■

Medicolegal Issues in Telephone Medicine

Malpractice cases that focus directly on telephone triage decisions and by whom telephone medicine advice is given are increasing. Based on an analysis of 6000 general risk management issues, the top four categories that were identified were clinical judgment, technical skill, communication, and documentation.[1] Communication and documentation have shown the greatest rate of increased claims over the past several years. In terms of liability and risk, telephone medicine does not differ from any other area of health care, although telephone triage has evolved into primarily a nursing specialty. The risk of a lawsuit involving the telephone is determined by the degree to which nurses and other health care professionals are specifically trained in telephone triage protocols and documentation and by the infrastructure of the systems in which they function.

Malpractice suits can be directed at the medical group or the medical care organization for not having a well-organized telephone triage system, against the involved clinician for a delay in diagnosis, or against the triage nurse for failure to follow established protocols.[2] As discussed in Chapter 1, most medicolegal problems can be traced to three root causes: poor documentation, lack of policies and protocols, and inadequate training of staff members.

Reducing Malpractice Liability

Several preventive measures can be taken to reduce liability and simultaneously improve the quality of care. Questions now routinely asked by attorneys in the event of a malpractice claim can serve as a checklist of how an office practice is functioning and highlight opportunities for improvement.

During questioning in a deposition, clinicians should be prepared to answer the following questions from the plaintiff's lawyer:

- Who took the call?
- What is that person's educational background?
- What has been the training in telephone triage, and by whom?
- What are the written policies and procedures for the practice?
- Whose protocols are used? (Not "**Are** protocols used?")
- Did the triage person consult with you about the call?
- Show me the telephone log documenting the call (or calls).
- Do you review the telephone triage encounters every day?

The defense response may be, "The call came from someone who was unknown and had never been seen before in our office. She had a cough with high fever and the office nurse simply referred her to the local emergency room for care."

Liability is based on whether a clinician-patient relationship existed.[3] Patients do not have to be seen or examined in order to establish this kind of relationship if the court can be convinced that the telephone conversation constituted treatment. If the caller was told, and this was documented, that "our office refers all new patient contacts for acute problems to the local emergency room for care," most would agree that no patient-clinician relationship was established and therefore no liability existed. However, if a medical history was taken and the caller was told, "Your symptoms suggest the possibility of pneumonia, and we advise you to go to the local emergency room," a relationship may have been created—contrary to the intent—that most likely had imposed a legal obligation. This relationship, which determines liability, can be explicit, implicit, or imposed by the court. The plaintiff must then establish that a breach in the standards of care occurred (cause) that resulted in an injury (damages). This sequence—relationship, deviation from standards of care, and a resulting adverse outcome—is the core of a malpractice suit.

As a key step in reducing liability, all medically significant calls should be carefully documented and retained as part of the patient's medical record. A telephone encounter form is recommended for most practices. Formats vary, ranging from portable pocket-sized pads for after-hours use to log books and self-adhesive sticker forms that can be entered into the record. Computerized systems are also available for real-time chart entry, but such programs are expensive. A sample of the basic information that should be recorded for all calls is listed in Table 3–1.

Case Illustration: The Importance of Good Documentation

The importance of good documentation is illustrated by a case in which a Midwest jury found a medical group negligent based solely on the advice given to parents by a registered nurse.[4] The nurse was employed by a highly regarded pediatric group, which offered a nurse counseling service as an enhancement to their practice. In this case, a pediatrician had diagnosed "flu" in a little girl during an office visit. The parents called 36 hours later to report on her progress and request advice. The parents remembered stating that their child was much worse, irritable, and listless. The nurse offered an appointment, and the parents admitted in their deposition that they declined

---

TABLE 3–1 Basic Information to Be Recorded for Each Telephone Encounter

Identifying Information:
    Name, age, home telephone, and patient ID or health plan number
    Identity of caller and relationship to patient
Chief complaint or purpose of call
Outcome of call
    Appointment advised and accepted
    Call referred to (specify)
    Follow-up instructions
    Consulted with (specify)
Home management advice and treatment (specify)
Message for clinician to call patient back
    Nature of problem and urgency
    How soon patient expects the call

it. The actual log was retrieved 10 years later, photographically enlarged and displayed boldly on the courtroom wall facing the jurors. Words such as "fussy," "listless," and "temperature" were recorded in such a way that they could have meant anything. The nurse could not recall the case. There was nothing in the log about the declined appointment. The plaintiff's lawyers had a field day. The plaintiff was awarded 2.5 million dollars.

> When the lawyers for the defense were asked why the case was lost, they replied that no documentation would have been better than the way in which the telephone log, retrievable after 10 years, portrayed the encounter. The fact that an appointment was offered should have been clearly documented. Further, ambiguous words such as "listless" and "irritable" are open to interpretation and convey that the patient should have been seen, or at the least, the supervising physician, who was in the office at the time, should have been made aware of the situation. This should have been documented as "Dr. consulted." If the patient refuses any advice or recommendation, this should be clearly documented on the telephone encounter form.

Case Illustration: Red Light Alert— Multiple Calls for Continuing Symptoms

A 35-year-old engineer became ill with diarrhea and fever the day after his return from a 3-day business trip to Mexico. When he developed a temperature of 104°, sore throat, and dry cough, he was seen by his physician in an urgent care center. The diagnosis was acute pharyngitis, possibly streptococcal. A throat culture was obtained and the patient was started on oral penicillin treatment. The following day his wife called for the throat culture results and reported that her husband still had a fever. The receptionist told her that the throat culture results were pending and that it was not unusual for the fever to persist for a few days.

The wife called a second time because her husband seemed worse, was coughing more and complained of some tightness in his chest. She was told to continue treatment. That night, in response to a third call at 9:30 P.M., the triage nurse spoke to the physician. The nurse told the patient's wife that she had consulted with the doctor, who said it was not unusual to have fever for several days; her husband should drink fluids and stay on the penicillin. The throat culture result was due in the morning.

The patient did not speak with the doctor as his wife requested. In the morning the patient went directly to another physician and was admitted to the hospital in respiratory failure with Legionnaire's disease. Angry because her husband was not given an appointment after several calls, the patient sued the nurse, physician, and urgent care center for negligence. The physician had no recollection of being consulted, although it was noted by the nurse in the telephone log.

> Whenever a patient calls back because symptoms either are not improving or are getting worse, the antennae for a visit should be raised. There should be no decrease in the intensity of questioning just because the patient was previously seen in the office—instead, the intensity of questioning should be increased. How the triage nurse is expected to address this problem should be clearly defined by the supervising physician. In some cases it will automatically indicate a visit; in other situations the nurse will be directed to consult the physician, who may wish to speak directly to the patient.

Case Illustration: Practice Good Medicine First

A 44-year-old man experienced chest pain suggestive of angina while mowing the lawn on a hot summer day. He and his wife thought it was heartburn from the pasta he had eaten for lunch. They belonged to an HMO and called the urgent care center. The triage nurse advised his wife to take him to the hospital as stated in the HMO's policy book and gave her directions to the hospital with which they had a contract. The HMO's hospital was 15 miles away. The patient collapsed en route and was dead on arrival. The nearest hospital was 5 minutes from the patient's home; he passed it on the way to the HMO's hospital. In addition, the patient was not advised to call an ambulance. The case was settled out of court.

> Patients should always be directed to go to the nearest hospital by ambulance whenever there is a possibility of a life-threatening emergency. A managed care contract with a hospital should never influence the decision to get to the nearest hospital in a life-threatening emergency situation.

Maintaining Patient Confidentiality

The sensitivity surrounding patient confidentiality and the associated risks of liability for breaches of confidentiality have never been greater. The concern about privacy and unauthorized access to patient information is heightened by the increasing use of computerized medical records. Psychiatric histories, diagnoses (such as HIV) that could be damaging to employment opportunities, and information about pregnancy and sexually transmitted disease in the adolescent population are examples of exquisitely sensitive information that should be guarded against any breach of confidentiality and never handled in casual manner, such as being left as a message on an answering machine. The guiding principle should be to never divulge any information about a patient without written consent from either the patient or the patient's guardian—to employers, insurance companies, schools, relatives, or health departments.[5]

An additional concern is the way in which confidential telephone conversations occur in many offices within the earshot of other patients and staff. If at all possible, these conversations should take place in telephone rooms or areas separated from the waiting room or reception area. The use of fax machines, cellular telephones, and e-mail pose an additional threat to patient confidentiality. The risks associated with electronic transmission of medical information should not be underestimated. Electronic communication tools should be considered as confidential as the medical record itself. For example, medical information should be faxed only if the patient consents and all measures are taken to ensure confidentiality. Cases and patient information should never be discussed over cellular telephones.

Summary: Steps to Reduce Risk in Telephone Medicine

- Documentation should be smarter, not longer.
- Avoid ambiguous terms such as "listless," "fussy," or "irritable," which are open to interpretation.
- If there is a **second call** for the same problem, the physician either should be consulted or should speak directly with the patient.
- If there are **three calls** for a persisting or worsening problem, the patient should be seen.

- Protocols and decision guidelines are essential.
- Document any patient noncompliance (e.g., if an appointment or advice is refused).
- Triage decisions should not be influenced by managed care contracts if safety is a concern. (For example, if an emergency is suspected, direct the patient to the nearest hospital, regardless of any HMO contract.)
- Regular review and evaluations of the quality of telephone medicine performance and service by staff should be integrated into the triage system and documented.

REFERENCES

1. Risk Management Foundation Quarterly. Harvard Medical Institutions, Cambridge, MA, Fall 1998.
2. Wick, W, and Katz, HP: Telephone contracts and counseling. In American College of Legal Medicine (ed): Legal Medicine, ed 3. Mosby-Year Book, St. Louis, 1995, pp 343–350.
3. Howard, ML, and Vogt, LB: Physician-patient relationship. In American College of Legal Medicine (ed): Legal Medicine, ed 3. Mosby-Year Book, St. Louis, 1995, pp 265–273.
4. Katz HP: Malpractice, meningitis, and the telephone. Pediatric Annals Feb:85–98, 1991.
5. Telephones and electronic technology (Questions 31–39). In 100 Questions about Health Care Risk Management. Risk Management Foundation of the Harvard Medical Institutions, Cambridge, MA, 1996, pp 31–39.

TELEPHONE SKILLS IN PRIMARY HEALTH CARE

Harvey P. Katz, MD

CHAPTER 4

The Art of Telephone Medicine

The office or clinic staff members who are selected for telephone responsibility are the vital link between clinicians and anyone calling the office—patients, vendors, colleagues, and hospitals. Professional telephone etiquette is an essential communication skill for everyone in the office who uses the telephone. Because these staff members will create the image and voice of the practice, they will profoundly influence quality of care, patient and practitioner satisfaction, and the growth of the practice. The wrong person in this sensitive position can spell disaster.

> A major objective of training is for all telephone staff to have a heightened sense of their importance every time they answer the phone.

What is "the art of telephone medicine"? It is developing a "phoneside manner" much like a clinician's bedside manner. For example, when the art is poorly executed, callers can receive exactly what they ask for—such as an appointment—but nevertheless can be made to feel angry or upset: angry over the manner in which they were spoken to or upset by the negotiations they were put through, as if the staff member was doing them a great favor by "working them in." Patients do not need to hear how busy the clinician is or that he or she is at lunch! On the other hand, callers who don't get what they ask for can still end up extremely satisfied with the outcome: "Your doctor is not available (or is at the hospital) this morning, but I know she would love to see you herself this afternoon, rather than have anyone else see you. . . . Is there a time this afternoon that would be convenient for you?" This ability is the "art." Some people are naturals. Most require training and must learn to develop the right mindset, which says, "Treat the patient as you would like to be treated if you were on the other end of the phone." This is the golden rule of telephone medicine.

The first, key step in developing a telephone care program is to hire the right person. Individuals selected for the telephone at all levels—secretary, receptionist, medical assistant, registered nurse, nurse practitioner, or physician assistant—must be carefully recruited and trained. Physicians also should be trained in telephone practices. In addition to basic knowledge, other qualifications should include warmth and compassion, intelligence, sound judgment, and excellent language and communication skills. Diversity among staff is an enhancement if personnel are bilingual for specific populations such as Hispanic or Asian. Telephone medicine responsibilities should be discussed in detail during the applicant's interview to emphasize its importance and to evaluate the applicant's telephone skills.

In most settings a nurse is selected for the telephone medicine responsibility because of prior clinical training and because medicolegal liability will be less than if nonclinical personnel are used. Many clinicians have employed specially trained, non-nurse health assistants, either alone or in combination with a nurse triage specialist. The extent of teaching and supervision that will be necessary depends on the degree of responsibility the practitioner wishes to delegate; the knowledge base, experience, motivation, and style of the telephone staff person; and the characteristics of the population served.

Telephone Style: Your Voice Creates the Image

When using the telephone, **your voice is you.** The patient can't see you and you can't see the patient. Be expressive and put the punctuation into your voice—the ??? and the !!!. It is helpful to tape record your greeting to patients and then listen to yourself to evaluate whether your speech is clear, with a normal tone, and at a moderate rate and if you have an appropriate level of animation in your voice.

Experienced triage nurses know that patients are quick to sense the desire to help, and if that is combined with empathic, sound advice, even the most difficult patient will be understanding and cooperative. If the patient is upset and angry, the triage rule is not to argue. If necessary, transfer the call to the clinician along with all the available background information. The art of managing the upset, irate patient is discussed later in this chapter.

Other helpful suggestions for staff to start the telephone caller on the right foot include:

- **Answer the telephone promptly.** Ringing telephones are a major source of irritation to everyone. Set a goal of picking up the telephone after no more than three rings. If the telephone system has automatic call distribution (ACD), which puts patients in a queue, set the goal of breaking into the machine voice for at least 90% of the calls.
- **Avoid the "Is this an emergency, may I put you on hold?—Click" syndrome.** Always allow the patient to respond. If you must leave the caller for a moment, explain and ask, "Will you please stay on the line while I check that information?" or ". . . while I get the doctor?" If it takes more than a minute, offer to call back if you can. When you do return to the line, thank the caller for waiting.
- **Go the extra mile.** If you cannot provide the information, offer to find someone who can solve the problem. When you are overloaded, there is always the useful option of taking down the number and calling back.

TABLE 4-1	**What's Your Courtesy Quotient?**

1. Do you identify yourself properly and show that you will take responsibility for the call?
2. Do you use the caller's name and give your full attention to the call?
3. Do you answer promptly and greet callers pleasantly? Do you put "Good morning" and "How may I be of help" into your voice?
4. Do you take notes to avoid having the caller repeat information?
5. Do you apologize for delays?
6. Do you treat callers as if they were a good friend or close relative?
7. When you promise a callback, do you follow through?
8. Do you place calls as courteously and efficiently as you like to receive them yourself?

- **Be discreet, confidential, and sensitive.** When a caller is upset, there is always a reason, but it usually is unknown. For example, there may have been a recent death in the family or the parent may have been up all night with a crying infant. Here is where listening skills and a caring attitude are critical.

These basic principles may be forgotten in the heat of a busy day, when the telephone never stops ringing. We are all human. Some need reminding more than others. Telephone triage staff can perform a self-evaluation by answering the questions in Table 4–1. A high score indicates proficiency in the art of telephone medicine.

The Anatomy of a Telephone Encounter

The telephone encounter, while complex, has a skeleton consisting of three basic parts:

- Greeting or "verbal handshake"
- Obtaining the history or the relevant information to make the triage decision
- Closure by making a disposition or offering help

The Four-Part Greeting

The greeting or "verbal handshake" sets the tone for the encounter and should be pleasant and professional. The four parts include:

1. Friendly introduction such as "Good morning"
2. Identification of the department to make sure callers know they have connected with the right place: "Department of . . ." or "This is Dr. Myers' office."
3. Name: "I'm Ms. Johnson."
4. The offer of help: "How may I be of help?"

Ideally all four points should be used. When the telephone gets too busy, the four points can be abbreviated to save time. Anyone who talks to patients on the telephone can improve his or her style and tone by practicing into a tape recorder in order to achieve a greeting that comes across as professional and caring.

There is a significant difference between "Good afternoon, this is Chris—may I be of help?" versus a cold, "Hello, Internal Medicine." Try the verbal handshake with erect posture versus slouching with the face held downward and with and without a smile in your voice. Note the difference. Good posture and the appropriate affect create a communication style that establishes immediate rapport with the patient. This is necessary for obtaining an accurate history. It stands in for the handshake and greeting in the exam room.

The History

The second part, obtaining the necessary information to make a relevant disposition, requires skill in history taking (see Chapter 5), experience, and concentration. The telephone encounter is considerably more difficult than a face-to-face visit. The pace is faster, visual clues are absent, and distractions—noise, patient traffic, and multiple interruptions to do other things—are everywhere.

The telephone assistant has to rely on tone and expression, how questions are phrased, and a careful choice of words. Questions can be either closed or open ended. Both types have their place in history taking. An example of a closed-ended, or directive, question is "Does it hurt when you move the arm?" This will elicit a Yes or No answer and saves time. An open-ended, or nondirective, question would be asked as "Can you tell me how it feels, or what the pain is like?" Although it takes more time, patients should be permitted to express their concerns in order to get the history that is most accurate and relevant to the reason for the call. The experienced telephone assistant can help guide even the most rambling, vague patient history by combining an assertive style, being knowledgeable, and knowing when it is appropriate to ask closed versus open questions.

Disposition

The third part of the telephone encounter closes the loop by offering advice and help. The disposition can be of four types:

1. An appointment for the patient to be seen
2. A message for someone else to return the call
3. Referral to another source, such as a department, person, specialty area, or local emergency room
4. Home management advice and follow-up instructions

Once a solution has been offered for a problem, it is critical that all efforts should be made to follow through and honor the offer. Always do what has been promised. For example, if the disposition is for someone to call back within an hour, someone should do so. Nothing causes more anger and frustration than for a patient not to receive a call that is promised or for it to be late. Conversely, confidence is enhanced if the call is on time. Achieving this result not only depends on an efficient telephone staff but also requires a smooth-functioning office message system and the cooperation of all clinicians.

Managing the Upset or Angry Patient

The ultimate challenge to the telephone medicine specialist is managing an irate, upset patient. Fortunately, these patients are encountered only rarely, but when they are, the encounter can be devastating to the inexperienced telephone assistant who, while trying to do his or her best to help, finds the encounter out of control. Training, experience, and advance preparation for managing this specific type of problem are essential. If telephone assistants can keep their cool, separate the person from the situation, solve the problem, and turn the angry patient into a loyal and appreciative friend, they have mastered the art of telephone medicine. To help, here are eight tips:

1. **Don't take it personally.** Contrary to how it feels, the patient's anger is not directed at you personally. Upset patients are angry at situations over which they feel they have no control. It takes training and experience to stay calm, listen, and resist the reflex to react.
2. **Let the patient vent.** Even though it takes time, nothing we say sinks in while an angry patient is blowing off steam. A good strategy is to "hang out like the

TABLE 4-2 **Deadly Phrases**	
Don't Say:	*Try This Instead:*
"I disagree."	"I understand. Let's discuss the problem."
"Let's compromise."	"Let's find a solution by working together."
[The clinician . . .]	"The clinician is not available at this time. May I
"is on vacation"	take a message so that he/she or one of his/her
"is at lunch"	colleagues can call you back?"
"is busy—has no time in the schedule"	
"never works on Wednesday"	
"It's our policy."	"We recommend doing it this way because . . ."
"You have to . . ."	"Here is something you may wish to try because I think it will help."
"You missed your appointment last week because you came late."	"There may have been a misunderstanding about the appointment time. Let's see if we can work it out."

fog" (listening is therapeutic) and wait for the right opening. It always comes, sooner or later, and when it does, grab it out of the air. Anything that sounds positive is a great time to break in. For example, a patient may say, "I can't understand what's going on in that place, I always used to be given an appointment sooner." At that moment the patient is recalling a more positive experience from the past and may be ready to listen. You can respond, "You're right about that. We're sorry it didn't go as well this time. Let's work on getting you seen as soon as possible."

3. **Avoid deadly phrases.** Certain phrases only make angry patients angrier. See Table 4–2 for examples of phrases to avoid and more tactful replacements.

4. **Acknowledge feelings.** An excellent way to establish rapport is by using the technique of mirroring feelings, that is, paraphrasing in your own words how the person is feeling. Listen for a pause or break into the anger and respond, "I understand that you must be feeling frustrated. . . . Specifically, how can I help you?"

5. **Separate the person from the situation.** This will help you avoid the accuse–defend–reaccuse cycle. A patient may say, "You told me that the doctor would call," to which the answerer responds, "No I didn't," and then the caller comes back with "Yes, you most certainly did." The issue at hand is not discussed. Although it is difficult, always try to keep the central problem of the call in focus.

6. **Refer the call.** If you are getting nowhere, or if the call is consuming too much time while other patients are waiting, don't hesitate to ask your supervisor or the patient's clinician to help by speaking to the patient directly. Tell the patient that you will have someone call him or her back within a specific amount of time and move on to the next patient.

7. **Follow up.** The best way to turn an angry patient into an appreciative and loyal friend for the future is to do what you say you are going to do and then follow up on it. In some cases, making a return call to ensure that the follow-up plan has worked out satisfactorily may be an excellent investment of time for both staff and patient satisfaction. It demonstrates that you really do care.

8. **Take a break.** When it is all over, take a mental and physical time-out as a way of dealing with "phone stress." If the call turned out well, congratulate yourself on a job well done, and share the experience with others.

CHAPTER 5

■ ■ ■ ■ ■ ■ ■ ■ ■ ■ ■ ■ ■ ■
■
■
■
■
The Medical History

The most helpful part of the evaluation of any medical problem is the history, or narrative, of the illness. The physical examination usually confirms the history in establishing the proper diagnosis. The least important part of the evaluation is the use of laboratory tests.

> In the real world of a busy primary care practice, the keys to a good history are relevance (seeking the most important questions that yield the greatest amount of useful information), the ability to judge the relationship the clinician has with the patient and family as a means of assessing the validity and objectivity of the reported information, and, finally, the art of being a good listener—for both facts and feelings.

There is little time for a long, detailed discussion when several other patients are on hold, impatiently waiting to present their problems. Decisions have to be made quickly and accurately. Everyone being trained in history-taking experiences a case in which he or she spends a long time nervously taking the clinical history and performing a physical examination without gaining any real insight into the patient's problem. The attending clinician then walks in, puts the patient at ease within seconds, gently asks one or two probing questions (which the student somehow overlooked), and within minutes has the answer to the patient's problem. This is what is meant by relevance.

To save time and avoid errors, if a new patient whose medical and social background is unknown calls about an illness, an appointment should be made immediately. The same is true for someone who is agitated or whose language is difficult to understand.

Parts of the Medical History

The medical history is an objective way of learning as much as possible about the patients' symptoms and the factors that may be influencing the problem, and it can be an effective means of quickly assessing the needs of a patient in a telephone encounter. For triage staff, it may be helpful to review the components of a complete history as it is practiced by clinicians when the patient is seen in the office. The same general approach is applicable over the telephone.

> The component parts of a medical history include:
> - Chief complaint
> - History of the present illness
> - Review of systems
> - Past medical history, family history, and social history

Chief Complaint

The *chief complaint (CC)* is defined as the reason for the patient's call and the description of the problem, stated in the caller's own words. It is not a diagnosis. For example, "ear infection" is not a chief complaint when the parent actually said, "My child has an earache." The historian should note the chief complaint verbatim. Other examples of chief complaints might include "fever," "not feeling well," "failing in school," or "fussiness," "stomach ache," or "chest pain." It is important for the person answering the telephone to appreciate the specific reason why a patient is calling by practicing the art of listening. The chief complaint is the portion of the history that is the introduction to the other parts.

History of the Present Illness

The *history of the present illness (HPI)* is the patient's opportunity to detail the specifics that characterize the chief complaint. In an orderly fashion, the patient is encouraged to narrate the development, nature, and chronology of the symptoms as background to the chief complaint. As discussed in Chapter 4, knowing what kind of questions to ask is an art. Both closed- and open-ended questions have their place. With training and experience, the telephone assistant will learn to control the conversation appropriately.

The following examples illustrate how the history of the present illness provides the background for the chief complaint. Sometimes the historian will also search for associated symptoms using a review of systems and will ask about the past-, family-, and social-history components of the narrative, which are discussed later in this chapter.

CC: A 9-year-old complains of a stomachache.

HPI: The pain is dull and achy, started around the navel, and moved toward the lower right side of the abdomen. It began last night, steadily grew worse, and is now associated with fever of 102°F (rectal) and vomiting. The child has vomited twice in the past 2 hours and is now refusing to eat or drink. There have been no diarrhea or urinary tract symptoms.

QUICK ASSESSMENT: Possible surgical problem (?appendicitis).

PLAN: Immediate appointment

CC: The parent states that her 2-year-old has diarrhea.

HPI: In the past 2 days, the child has had eight watery bowel movements that do not contain blood or mucus. He is acting listless, has a temperature of 103°F, and has vomited once today. There has been no urine in the past 8 hours. Liquid nourishment is refused. The father had a similar illness 4 days ago and recovered without specific treatment.

QUICK ASSESSMENT: Possible dehydration.

PLAN: Immediate appointment.

CC: Fever of 102°F.

HPI: This 3-year-old girl has a slight runny nose but is otherwise alert and active. She is playful, and, although her appetite has fallen off a bit, she is drinking well. The cold has been present for the past 2 days and does not seem to be getting worse. She is not particularly fussy or lethargic.

QUICK ASSESSMENT: Probable minor illness.

PLAN: Home advice and follow-up instructions (e.g., fussiness may mean an ear infection).

CC: Wife says husband "says he has heartburn."

HPI: Wife reports that 46-year-old man was playing basketball with son. Suddenly developed pressure in chest that felt like heartburn. He had pizza for lunch. Chest feels heavy and sensation is now spreading down left inner arm and up into jaw. No prior heart disease.

QUICK ASSESSMENT: Possible heart attack.

PLAN: Activate EMS/911 system.

CC: "Sore throat"

HPI: 23-year-old woman awoke with a sore, scratchy throat 2 hours ago. No fever or other URI symptoms. Feels generally well. No exposure to strep.

QUICK ASSESSMENT: Sore throat of 2 hours duration; too early for specific explanation.

PLAN: Tylenol for pain if needed, more humidity in home. Call back if symptom worse after 24 hours or new symptoms develop.

Review of Systems

A *review of systems (ROS)* is a survey of all organ systems (head, eyes, ears, nose, throat, lungs, heart, abdomen, genitourinary system, and neurologic system). The survey should be relevant to the present illness; for instance, the parent of a child with a fever should be questioned about the genitourinary complaints of burning on urination or frequency of urination as a clue to the presence of a urinary tract infection. Many times callers will not offer this information spontaneously if their focus is on another symptom.

A brief review of systems fits quite naturally with the history of the present illness. The nature of the complaint will determine which systems should be surveyed and how extensively. For example, thorough questioning about neurologic symptoms is appropriate for a complaint of head trauma but is less relevant if the complaint is abdominal pain.

Past History, Family History, Social History

For the purpose of telephone medicine, the past history deals with any pertinent information about the patient's past that relates to the present illness. This would include information about previous serious illnesses, hospitalizations, or drug allergies, for instance, that bear on the present illness or may influence therapy. For example, a patient who has had a seizure is always questioned about any previous traumatic episode in which there may have been injury to the brain. It is important to know if a patient presenting with asthma has been hospitalized in the past, as a means of gauging the potential course of this attack. A child exposed to chickenpox will be managed quite differently if he or she is receiving cancer chemotherapy or steroid medication for kidney problems. These examples show the importance of always determining if there is any chronic underlying or coexisting disease.

In the same way that a past history provides meaningful information, so too do the family history and social history. A strong family history of diabetes, thyroid disease, or kidney disease may have a direct bearing on a child's illness. Social history includes sensitive information about family structure and substance abuse. It is inappropriate for telephone assistants to ask for details of this delicate and confidential history, however, which should be reserved for the privacy of an office visit. On the other hand, clues to the presence of a socially problematic situation are often picked up over the phone and should be relayed to the clinician who is scheduled to see the patient.

Potential Pitfalls

Errors in diagnosis can occur even when patients are examined by clinicians in the office, particularly when the symptoms are mild and the patient is seen very early in the course of the disease. The chances of error increase when large numbers of patients have to be handled quickly, as in the case of an influenza epidemic. Among hundreds of patients with similar symptoms, one with a different, more serious illness can slip by unnoticed. This rarely happens, but it is easy for health care providers to be lulled into a sense of false security by the large numbers of patients who have mild complaints. In such circumstances, it is wise to pause and reflect upon what else a patient could have, instead of jumping to a hasty conclusion. This is what is meant by "differential diagnosis." Most patients do have straightforward symptoms of a problem or illness that is usually mild. Life-threatening problems generally are not obscure, although an emergency is in the eye of the beholder. If there is any doubt about whether a patient should be seen, one should err on the side of safety. When the decision is to offer advice for home care, the door should always be left open for patients to call back if there is a significant change.

Tables 5–1 and 5–2 are presented to stimulate a heightened index of suspicion. They present serious conditions that might potentially be missed (in children and in adults), what the condition might be mistaken for, and the critical piece of the history that should tip off the telephone assistant that the patient should be seen because of the risk of a serious problem. In some circumstances, it may even be advisable to make alternative arrangements, such as calling 911 or an on-call clinician, if the patient's regular clinician is not "in." Avoiding pitfalls of this type is one of the aims of the Telephone Decision Guidelines that accompany Chapters 8 through 62.

In summary, one can view the parts of a history as components that should dovetail into a cohesive, logical picture of the patient's problem. The skills needed to accomplish this quickly and accurately over the telephone come with practice and experience.

TABLE 5-1 Potential Diagnostic Errors in Telephone History Taking: Pediatric

Serious Diagnosis that Could Be Missed	Benign Condition for Which It Might Be Mistaken	Possible Tip-off: The Critical History
Acute appendicitis	Gastroenteritis	Right-sided abdominal pain or any persisting or increasing abdominal pain
Anaphylaxis	Simple allergic reaction or hives	Difficulty swallowing or breathing; wheezing; generalized swelling; feeling dizzy with hives
Concussion or brain hemorrhage (subdural or epidural)	Minimal head trauma	Changes in behavior, personality, or mood after head trauma
Dehydration	Mild diarrhea	Lethargy, decreased urine output, no tears in infant
Epiglottitis	Mild croup	Fever, irritability, pain on swallowing; difficulty handling salivation (drooling)
Hypoglycemia (low blood sugar)	Unrelated illness or moodiness	Known diabetes, irrational behavior, drowsiness
Meningitis	Muscle spasm of neck	Extreme irritability and stiff neck
Meningococcemia	Benign viral rash	Petechiae (small hemorrhages into the skin); child appearing ill to parent
Rabies	Harmless bite from a wild animal	All bites from skunks, raccoons, bats are rabid until proven otherwise
Reye's syndrome	Gastroenteritis	Mental confusion with persistent vomiting (especially if associated with influenza or chickenpox)
Sepsis/meningitis	Mild URI with fever	Fever before age of 4 months
Severe drug overdose	Minimal ingestion	Amount of drug ingested is critical; ask how much is left in bottle or how many pills are left of original prescription
Testicular torsion	Pulled groin muscle	Testicular pain or swelling
Toxic shock syndrome	Gastroenteritis, diarrhea	Profuse watery diarrhea, faint rash, looks ill (teenager)

TABLE 5-2 Potential Diagnostic Errors in Telephone History Taking: Adult		
Serious Diagnosis that Could Be Missed	**Benign Condition for Which It Might Be Mistaken**	**Possible Tip-off: The Critical History**
Anaphylaxis	Simple allergic reaction or hives	Difficulty swallowing or breathing, wheezing, generalized swelling, feeling dizzy with hives
Appendicitis	Gastroenteritis	Localized right-sided or abdominal pain
Concussion or brain hemorrhage	Minimal head trauma	Changes in behavior, personality, or mood after head trauma
Diabetes	Urinary tract infection	Increased thirst and appetite with weight loss
Ectopic pregnancy	Gastroenteritis	Lower abdominal pain, a missed period, irregular vaginal bleeding
Hepatitis	Mild gastroenteritis	Dark urine and yellow sclera (white of the eye)
Hypoglycemia (low blood sugar)	Unrelated illness or moodiness	Known diabetes, irrational behavior, drowsiness
Meningitis	Muscle spasm of neck	Extreme irritability and stiff neck
Meningococcemia	Benign viral rash	Petechiae (small hemorrhages into the skin) and patient appearing ill
Myocardial infarction (heart attack)	Muscle strain or indigestion	Chest pain associated with sweating, lightheadedness, extreme anxiety, chest pressure, or jaw/arm pain
Rabies	Harmless bite from a wild animal	All bites from skunks, raccoons, bats are rabid until proven otherwise
Severe drug overdose	Minimal ingestion	Amount of drug ingested is critical; ask how much is left in bottle or how many pills are left of original prescription
Stroke or transient ischemic attack (TIA)	Benign dizziness, pins and needles feelings from sleeping or pressure on an arm or leg	**Sudden** weakness in an extremity, numbness on one side of face or body, dizziness, loss of vision, confusion, or difficulty speaking or understanding others
Testicular torsion	Pulled groin muscle	Testicular pain or swelling
Toxic shock syndrome	Gastroenteritis, diarrhea	Profuse, watery diarrhea; faint rash; patient looks ill

CHAPTER 6

Prescribing Medication Over the Telephone

When medicine is prescribed over the telephone, instructions must be clear and accurate to avoid any possibility of error. Always determine:

- If the patient has any known drug allergies
- If the patient is taking other medications (to prevent possible adverse drug interactions) and what amount is being given (to ensure appropriate dosage)
- If an appropriate medication (e.g., ibuprofen, acetaminophen, syrup of ipecac, antacid) is already in the home (to save time and money)

When patients telephone to report an illness, treatment has frequently already begun at home, either with medication or some home remedy. As part of the history of the present illness, the telephone assistant should ask if any medication has been given at home, and if so, the dose and whether it is working. If the treatment is working, it can be encouraged and continued with the supervising physician's approval.

Selection of Over-the-Counter Drugs

The common over-the-counter (OTC) drugs can be categorized as follows:

- Cough, cold, and allergy preparations
- Gastrointestinal agents
- Pain relievers and antifever medicines
- Skin and hair care
- Women's health products
- Vitamin and nutritional supplements

There are more than 100,000 OTC preparations on the market, but together they use fewer than 1000 active ingredients. The average cost of an OTC medicine in 1998 was $5, compared to $22 for a prescription drug.

In selecting OTC drugs, many patients rely on their pharmacist's recommendation, cost, the advice of a friend, or a favorable past experience with a drug. In general, OTC drugs provide only symptomatic relief and do not treat the underlying disease. They should be selected on the basis of safety, efficacy, and cost. Those that are mentioned in this book represent the authors' preferences for the specific symptoms discussed. Drug information on OTCs has been obtained from the manufacturer's recommendations. All dosage schedules included in this book should be carefully reviewed for accuracy and modified according to individual preference by the supervising clinician.

If the supervising clinician has approved specific drugs to be recommended to patients, a customized list for the practice should be developed and reviewed periodically. Drugs on the list may be selected from the chapters of this book, or the clinician may wish to substitute other drugs for some symptoms. Tables 6–1 and 6–2 provide samples of the form such a list may take. The triage staff should review the list and keep it handy. Some of the chapters in Sections Three and Four of this book also include advice on the selection and use of OTC drugs. Useful general references include the *PDR for Nonprescription Drugs and Dietary Supplements,* published annually, and the annual OTC supplement to *Pharmacy Times.*

Drug Dosages for Children

Accurate measurements are needed for both safety and effectiveness. Adding to possible confusion and error are the proliferation of forms in which many drugs are available. By a recent count there were 110 brands of products containing acetaminophen, either alone or in combination, and 24 brands of ibuprofen. Many of these OTC drugs are available in more than one form. Tylenol, for example, comes in concentrated drops (100 mg acetaminophen/mL but dispensed as 80 mg/0.8 mL), a liquid or elixir (32 mg/mL dispensed as 160 mg/5 mL), and chewable tablets (80 or 320 mg). Ibuprofen comes labeled as 100 mg/2.5 mL. Specific pediatric doses for each are listed in Chapter 18. Parents should be encouraged to obtain a dosage chart from their clinician such as the one given there and to read the labels on OTC drugs carefully.

Dosages of drugs for children should be based on weight, whenever possible, rather than age. For antifever medication, the optimal dose for acetaminophen is 15 mg/kg (33 mg/lb); for ibuprofen it is 10 mg/kg (22 mg/lb).

Prescription Refills

Each clinician and practice have their own policies about whether drugs are ever prescribed for patients who have not been seen in the office for this episode of illness. Telephone assistants of course will need to refer all such requests to the supervising clinician. The telephone staff should be fully aware of the general policies and protocols in the practice for managing specific symptoms, such as prescribing antifever medications, so that the safest advice and follow-up instructions are provided.

A large number of calls are received in every office for prescription refills. The role of the telephone assistant is to expedite the request. This can be done by obtaining drug names and prescription numbers, validating that prescriptions are refillable, and relaying the information to the clinician for final closure. In many states, the clinician can authorize a nurse to call in the refill to the pharmacy.

TABLE 6-1   Preferred OTC Drugs and Other Products: Pediatric

Cough, Cold, and Allergy

Indication	Drug	Dose	Notes
For colds			
For cough			
For allergy			

Gastrointestinal Agents

Indication	Drug	Dose	Notes
Antacid			
For constipation (stool softener)			
For lactose intolerance			

Pain Relievers and Antifever Medications

Drug	Product	Dose	Notes
Acetaminophen			
Ibuprofen			

Skin and Hair Care

Indication	Product	Dose	Notes
For acne			

TABLE 6-1 Preferred OTC Drugs and Other Products: Pediatric *(Continued)*

Skin and Hair Care

Indication	Product	Dose	Notes
For warts			
For poison ivy			
For chapped lips			
For superficial skin infection			
For diaper rash (nonfungal)			
For diaper rash (fungal)			
For dry skin (moisturizer)			
For lice			

Vitamins and Nutritional Supplements

Indication	Product	Dose	Notes
Multivitamin			
Nutritional supplement			

child or adult appears so listless or irritable that medical attention is sought immediately. Between these two extremes, it may be unclear whether or not an appointment is really indicated. Decision-making in this gray zone, and sometimes even in the extremes, varies from patient to patient. Sound, informed judgment and the ability to appropriately balance the benefits and the risks of home management for a given medical situation are required for the best decision making. Even the guidelines in this book should be adapted to the needs of the individual practice setting and the socioeconomic characteristics of the population being served. So the role of the telephone assistant is key.

Chapter Structure

Each chapter in Sections Three and Four deals with an individual symptom or symptom complex. Each is divided into three interrelated subsections:

1. General medical background information
2. Telephone Decision Guidelines
3. Advice

Background

The most common symptoms presented by phone to pediatric and adult primary care practices have been selected for discussion in these chapters. The more knowledgeable that staff members are about the most common problems affecting patients, the more effectively they will be able to make decisions about advising patients. For example, if a patient calls complaining of a sore throat but has no other symptoms, it is important to find out whether the problem is a group A beta-hemolytic strep throat or not. If the staff member answering the phone has this fact clearly in mind, he or she will be able to make a rapid and appropriate triage decision. Patients can very quickly assess whether the staff member they are speaking to is knowledgeable. If they have confidence in the person on the other end of the phone, patients are more likely to comply with triage judgments as well as with management advice and follow-up instructions.

The background information provided in this book has been adapted to primary care medicine and emphasizes the practical aspects necessary for informed triage decisions. It can be used as a reference when speaking to a caller, as well as for training.

Telephone Decision Guidelines

The Telephone Decision Guidelines have been formulated to guide the telephone staff in helping parents and patients decide whether and when to be seen by a clinician. The Guidelines suggest (1) questions to be asked and (2) whether—and how urgently—to see the clinician based on the response to each question. Questions have been prioritized and clustered so that those revealing emergencies that require the patient to activate the emergency medical system or to be seen immediately in the office are asked first.

The guidelines use a graphic key with five options for when a patient should be seen if it is decided that an appointment is necessary. These options are:

EMS (Activate EMS or 911 system)
2 (see ASAP, within 1 to 2 hours at the latest)
8 (see same day)
24–72 (see within 3 days)
72 + (see in 4 days or more)

These options are only guides and can be readily modified according to the preferences of individual clinicians or the circumstances of the patients and the practice.

In a busy practice it is not realistic to expect that all relevant questions will be asked for every complaint. In this book we focus on questions that directly influence telephone triage. Some clinicians want telephone attendants to record additional information about such things as medications already tried, associated symptoms, and whether the patient has a history of similar episodes. These clinicians believe that having the answers to such questions helps them to prioritize when confronted with multiple patients and makes their own note taking more efficient when they do see the patient. But often time does not permit the luxury of a complete history, nor is one always needed. When a patient and past history are well known, fewer questions will be necessary than for a new patient. Also, if the situation is a true emergency, time should not be spent on less important questions. The Telephone Decision Guidelines in the following chapters have been formatted to help achieve efficient and informed decision making in an office setting by properly trained staff, most often a triage nurse. They should be studied so that they become second nature through memory and experience.

> In cases where a triage decision cannot be made by the telephone attendant, the decision guidelines also serve the purpose of selectively collecting the most important information to present to the clinician for review and final disposition.

Advice

If the decision is that an office visit is not indicated, it is appropriate for the telephone assistant to give the caller advice about home management. This section of each chapter also may include first-aid advice for emergencies and advice on changes that indicate the need for follow-up.

Using These Chapters for Training

Another objective of this book is to serve as a guide to a structured training program for individuals entrusted with a telephone medicine responsibility. Sections One and Two have provided a context for both supervisors and trainees. Sections Three and Four should be studied thoroughly by each telephone assistant as part of training and orientation. The decision guidelines can be used as the basis for role-playing sessions in which the supervising clinician or triage nurse assumes the role of patient or parent. These sessions can be a one-on-one exercise or can take place in a group discussion format between junior and senior staff assistants. A key element of training is for less experienced staff to observe and listen (perhaps on a two-way telephone setup) as the senior telephone-triage nurses are working.

Structured training in telephone medicine is applicable to many types of health professionals with a wide-ranging skill mix. Triage nurses are becoming more prevalent, but physicians, house staff, and medical assistants all could benefit from additional experience and training in telephone medicine. These chapters may help them to adopt a systematic approach in both learning and teaching about working with patients who call on the telephone.

SECTION THREE

TELEPHONE TRIAGE: SYMPTOMS IN CHILDREN

Harvey P. Katz, MD

CHAPTER 8

Abdominal Pain

Abdominal pain ranks high on the list of middle-of-the-night calls from frightened parents, preceded only by fever, earaches, and asthma. When children say their stomach hurts, parents immediately think of appendicitis. Because this possibility always exists, a thorough history should always focus on whether a surgical problem may be present. There are countless other causes of abdominal pain in children, so it is important to consider the diagnostic possibilities, particularly as they relate to the child's age.

Young Children (Less Than 2 Years Old)

It is best for all young children with the complaint of abdominal pain to be examined, chiefly because they are unable to verbalize their symptoms. Abdominal pain in young children can be caused by stomach virus infections, food allergy, urinary tract infections, pneumonia, sickle cell disease, and not uncommonly, constipation. The probability of a surgical problem, such as intestinal obstruction (e.g., intussusception), is increased when the parent reports that the knees are jackknifed (drawn up onto the chest) or if the child appears pale and sweaty. Frequently, when the parent reports that the infant appears to have a stomachache, something else may be present, such as an ear infection. This is another reason why young children should be given an appointment rather than home advice. In infants, frequent cycles of crying may represent colic and require an office visit for evaluation.

Older Children (Over 2 Years Old)

The diagnostic possibilities in older children are best divided into those of either chronic or acute/short duration. If abdominal pain has persisted for months (chronic), a future appointment is indicated. At that time, a detailed history and examination will be done to determine the cause, which can range from less common serious gastrointestinal disorders, like inflammatory bowel disease (Crohn's disease) and ulcers, to one of the most common causes of pain—anxiety and tension (functional or psychogenic). Stress-induced symptoms are often related to school or family dysfunction.

The most common cause of acute, nonlocalized abdominal pain is an intestinal viral infection, or gastroenteritis.

> The location of the pain in the description is very important, because any pain localized to the lower right side should be considered to be acute appendicitis until proved otherwise. The possibility of appendicitis must also be ruled out for any severe, generalized abdominal pain.

The typical history (and many cases are not typical) for appendicitis starts when the child loses his or her appetite at about the same time that stomach pain appears. Pain usually appears around the belly button, then travels to the right lower side. Low-grade fever, nausea, and vomiting are accompanying symptoms. It is important to be aware that some cases of appendicitis are caused by and often follow an acute gastroenteritis. Other causes of abdominal pain in older children include hepatitis (inflammation of the liver), a twisted ovary in girls, a blow to the abdomen in a sports contest or accident, and pneumonia. In adolescents, venereal disease (e.g., gonorrhea) should be suspected.

Another common, often overlooked, cause of abdominal pain is lactose (milk sugar) intolerance. Even small quantities of milk or milk solids in baked goods can cause gas and crampy abdominal pain.

In most instances of abdominal pain, home advice should not take the place of an examination. Once the clinician has established the diagnosis of a nonsurgical problem, follow-up care can be augmented by sound telephone management, focusing on the significance of changes in the child's condition and relief of symptoms.

TELEPHONE DECISION GUIDELINES

ABDOMINAL PAIN

Question	To See Clinician If . . .	When
1. Patient's name, telephone number, age, other identifying information	Under 3 years of age.	2
2. How severe is the pain? Is the child crying?	Severe, regardless of duration.	2
3. Was there any accident in which the stomach area was hurt?	Yes.	2
4. Where is the pain located?	On right side of abdomen.	2
5. Is the child acting particularly ill? Is the child playing or just lying around?	Yes, child appears ill, has fussiness, vomiting, pallor, sweating, or is lethargic.	2
6. Are there any associated symptoms?		
• Fever?	Over 103°F or fever has been present longer than 24 hours. See Chapter 18, Fever.	2
• Vomiting	Yes.	2
• Diarrhea	See Chaper 15, Diarrhea	8
• Difficulty breathing?	Yes.	2
• Severe cough or other chest symptoms?	Yes.	2
7. Is the pain constant or intermittent?	Constant.	2
8. Is the pain getting better or worse, or is it about the same?	Worse or the same.	8
9. Do any other family members have similar abdominal pain, vomiting, or diarrhea?	Yes.	8
10. How long has pain been present?	More than 48 hours (not severe).	24-72
11. What is the child's usual state of health?	Child has any chronic or serious condition (e.g., diabetes, asthma, cystic fibrosis, UTI).	8
12. Has the child been seen in the past for this problem?	Yes, complaint is chronic.	24-72

EMS = Activate EMS SYSTEM   24-72 = Appointment within 3 days

2 = See ASAP (within 1–2 hours)   72+ = Appointment in 4 days or more

8 = See same day

High priority items appear in color.

ADVICE

- If the infant is under 2 months old and has symptoms of colic, an appointment with the clinician is important. Once the diagnosis has been established, subsequent phone calls are best referred to the primary care clinician because parents may become extremely distraught and need direct access to the clinician who knows the family best.
- If symptoms of gastroenteritis are present and the pain is crampy, intermittent, and not severe or worsening, the child over 3 years of age can be observed at home and put on a clear liquid diet (see Chapter 15, Diarrhea), with instructions to call back if the pain increases or localizes to any specific area of the abdomen.
- If the pain is intermittent and crampy and there has been exposure to a similar illness at home, which includes vomiting, diarrhea, or both, the child can be observed at home. A clear liquid diet should be prescribed for 24 hours. If the child is hungry, dry toast or saltine crackers can be tried. The parent should call back if child is worse or symptoms change.

CHAPTER 9

▪ ▪ ▪ ▪ ▪ ▪ ▪ ▪ ▪ ▪ ▪ ▪ ▪ ▪
▪
▪
▪
Animal Bites
▪

The potential hazards of animal bites include infection with rabies, tetanus, and other bacterial agents causing local skin infections and the emotional trauma to the child as a result of the frightening experience.

Rabies

Rabies is an acute viral infection that spreads via peripheral nerves into the brain, causing a highly fatal brain infection (encephalitis). The rabies virus is transmitted in the infected saliva of a biting, warm-blooded animal. Over 40 species of animals in the world can be infected with rabies. The state health department can supply specific information about which animals have been infected with rabies in any given location, along with a detailed report of the types and number of animal bites for that state. These lists are very useful in describing the extent of the animal-bite problem in any given area. Data are usually categorized according to bites by common pets (cats, dogs, hamsters, rabbits); agricultural animals (horses, calves); primates (monkeys); wild rodents (chipmunks, ground hogs, mice, rats, squirrels); wild animals (bats, ferrets, raccoons, skunks); amphibians and reptiles (snakes, turtles, alligators), and miscellaneous animals such as spiders, camels, and crabs. In most instances, rodent bites can be assumed to be free of the threat of rabies.

Fortunately, human infection with rabies is rare. Symptoms can occur in as short as 3 days or as long as 6 to 9 months, depending on the amount of virus introduced into the wound (i.e., the extent of the bite) and the abundance of nerve supply at the wound site.

Some animals can transmit the disease at a time when they are not showing any symptoms. Rabies virus can be present in a dog's saliva for 2 to 7 days before the dog shows symptoms, and bats can be infected for more than a year without developing signs of illness. When dogs develop symptoms of rabies, death usually occurs in 4 to 5 days, making the 10-day observation period a valuable component of management.

All bat bites should be considered as an exposure to rabies. The diagnosis of rabies is based on specific laboratory tests performed on brain and salivary gland tissue of the animal, together with a clinical evaluation of the biting animal and the circumstances surrounding the incident. The prompt apprehension and careful observation of the biting animal is mandatory.

If bats, skunks, raccoons, and other wild animals are not captured, they must be assumed to be rabid.

Pet vaccination and animal-control programs are of the utmost importance for effective rabies prevention. Fortunately, there is a new rabies vaccine for humans that is safer, more effective, and requires many fewer injections than the older vaccine.

P
E
D
I
A
T
R
I
C

Local Skin Infections

Local skin infections can be prevented by prompt, thorough cleansing of the wound with soap and water. If the wound is extensive or deep, an appointment for an examination should be given as soon as possible.

Tetanus Immunization

After an animal bite or a cut, the risk of tetanus (lockjaw) is present, so the child's immunization status should be reviewed. The primary series of tetanus shots for a child consists of four doses, the last dose usually given at the 18-month well-baby visit. A booster dose is administered between 4 and 6 years of age and then every 10 years. A tetanus shot is advised following an animal bite if:

- More than 10 years have passed since the last immunization.
- More than 5 years have passed since the last shot and the wound is very dirty and contaminated.
- The child is under 6 years old and has not finished the complete four-dose series.
- The child has never been immunized. (In this case the entire series should be completed.)

TELEPHONE DECISION GUIDELINES

ANIMAL BITES

Question	To See Clinician If . . .	When
1. Patient's name, telephone number, age, other identifying information		
2. What kind of animal bit the child? Was it a wild animal or household pet?	Bat, skunk, fox, raccoon, monkey.	2
3. Was the bite unprovoked, or was the child playing with the animal?	Unprovoked bites by wild animals that would normally shy away from human contact are at highest risk for rabies.	2
4. How severe is the injury? Where are the bites?	Large lacerations requiring sutures; bites that appear infected; lacerations of the face or hand.	2
5. If the animal was a pet, has it been immunized for rabies?	No.	8
6. When did the bite occur? Is the animal available for observation?	If the animal cannot be located within a few hours, the child should be brought in and the circumstances reviewed by the clinician.	8
7. Has the child been immunized for tetanus? How long ago?	No, series incomplete or no shot within 10 years.	8

EMS = Activate EMS SYSTEM		24-72 = Appointment within 3 days
2 = See ASAP (within 1–2 hours)		72+ = Appointment in 4 days or more
8 = See same day		

High priority items appear in color.

A D V I C E

- Every effort should be made to locate the animal so that its health may be determined. The health department (or police if after hours) should be notified about animal bites so that appropriate investigation may be made. (Pets will not be taken away from their owners because of such a report.)

Telephone #: _____
County Health Department (fill in phone number)

Nights and Weekends #: _____
Police Department

- If the skin is not broken or if there is just a scratch, the wound should be thoroughly cleaned with soap and water and observed for infection.
- Uninfected bites by small household pets such as mice, hamsters, and gerbils generally are not at risk for rabies and need not be seen. The same advice applies for most rodents, including squirrels.

CHAPTER 10

■■■■■■■■■■■■■■
■
■
■
■
■

Asthma

Asthma is the most common chronic disease of childhood. The hallmarks of asthma are inflamed and hyper-reactive air passages (bronchioles) in the lungs. Asthma is also often referred to by other names, such as bronchial asthma, asthmatic bronchitis, reactive airway disease, bronchitis, and wheezy bronchitis.

An asthma attack can be triggered by allergies, exercise, colds, cigarette smoke, and changes in air quality. During an asthma attack, the inflamed lining of the airways develops bronchospasm, increased mucus production, and edema (swelling), leading to narrowing of the air passages. Two of the most common triggers are viral upper respiratory illness and exercise. Attacks during sports can be prevented if children prone to such attacks use a medication inhaler (e.g., albuterol) 15 minutes before exercise, as discussed later.

The first signs of an asthmatic attack are usually coughing, a feeling of tightness in the chest, shortness of breath, and classically a wheezing or whistling sound as the child breathes **out**. In contrast, croup (Chapter 14) usually sounds like a seal barking or a foghorn and occurs when the child breathes **in**. Most calls will come from parents of children known to have asthma. To gauge whether an appointment or medication adjustment is needed, ask what treatment has been tried at home, how the medication is working, and how this episode compares to previous attacks.

Asthma is highly variable and individual treatment plans are tailored to minimize or eliminate chronic symptoms. The severity of asthma can be graded according to the number of days and nights symptoms occur, as shown on Table 10–1.

Inhaled anti-inflammatory agents (cromolyn or an inhaled topical steroid such as beclomethasone [Beclovent]) are the most effective long-term control medication for asthma.

Asthma symptoms can be controlled with drugs (e.g., albuterol [Proventil]) given by inhaler or nebulization by machine (Fig. 10–1), either alone or combined with an anti-inflammatory drug. For optimal effect, these inhalers should be used with a spacer (for children over 5 years), or a mask if necessary. The spacer is a small plastic holding chamber that is connected to the inhaler (Fig. 10–2). It holds the medication so that it can be inhaled slowly, allowing it to penetrate the airways more effectively. It also reduces the bad taste and the possibility of thrush, a fungal infection of the membranes of the mouth, which appears as a thick, whitish coating.

If asthma is like a fire, "reliever" medication such as albuterol puts out the fire; "preventer" medication like inhaled steroids or cromolyn prevents the fire from starting. In moderate to severe asthma, both medications are needed in combination.

TABLE 10-1	Grades of Asthma Severity		
Grade	Days with Symptoms	Nights with Symptoms	Treatment
Mild intermittent asthma	≤ 2/week	≤ 2/month	Short-acting bronchodilator (albuterol) as needed; may not require daily medications
Mild persistent asthma	3–6/week	3–4/month	Short-acting bronchodilator as needed; inhaled anti-inflammatory (cromolyn or Tilade) or steroid (Beclovent) as preventive measure
Moderate persistent asthma	Daily	> 4/month	Inhaled anti-inflammatory steroid (Beclovent) and long-acting bronchodilator (salmeterol); short-acting bronchodilator as needed
Severe persistent asthma	Continual	Frequent	Inhaled anti-inflammatory, long-acting bronchodilator, and perhaps new leukotriene modifiers; short-acting bronchodilator as needed

A peak flow meter records the fastest speed at which the patient can blow air out of the lungs. Often, the rate of air flow decreases before wheezing is audible. Ask whether the patient has a peak flow meter and how today's reading compares with the "personal best." Most children over the age of 5 can learn how to use the meter accurately. If used, the goal is to keep the peak flow at or above 80% of the patient's

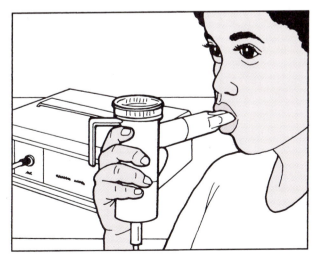

FIGURE 10-1 A nebulizer ("mist machine") for administering drugs to patients with asthma. (From *One Minute Asthma: What You Need to Know*, ed. 3. Thomas F. Plaut, M.D., Pedipress, Inc., Amherst, MA, 1996, p 37, with permission.)

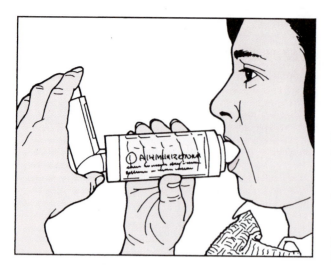

FIGURE 10-2 A holding chamber, also called a **spacer,** helps patients with asthma to use their inhaler more effectively. (From *One Minute Asthma: What You Need to Know,* ed. 3. Thomas F. Plaut, M.D., Pedipress, Inc., Amherst, MA, 1996, p 34, with permission.)

personal best score. Individual treatment plans can be created according to the peak flow readings and organized around color coded zones:

- **Green Zone.** Scores between 80 and 100 % of best score indicate good control. Patients should take their preventive anti-inflammatory medication.
- **Yellow Zone.** Scores between 50 and 80 % of best score are in the caution zone. Beta agonists such as albuterol should be started. Triggers should be avoided whenever possible. The clinician may want to prescribe a medication change. If the patient does not improve, an office appointment is indicated.
- **Red Zone.** A score less than 50 % of best peak flow is in the danger zone. **An immediate visit to either an emergency room or the office is indicated.**

Patient and parent education is critical, and if needed, an appointment should be made to review the treatment plan. Children with mild persistent asthma should be seen every 6 months for a progress review. If symptoms are minimal and the patient and parent are agreeable, home management is appropriate. If the asthma is worsening in spite of inhaled medication from either the nebulizer or metered-dose inhaler (MDI), or if mild, low-grade symptoms are not clearing after 3 to 4 days, the child should be seen in the office.

TELEPHONE DECISION GUIDELINES

ASTHMA

Question	To See Clinician If . . .	When
1. Patient's name, age, other identifying information		
2. Is the child wheezing, coughing, or both? Have you been told in the past that he/she has asthma?	Yes: See following questions. If not previously diagnosed as having asthma, go to question 9.	
3. Is the child having trouble breathing? Has medication been used?	Yes, poor color or lips blue. Struggling and straining to breathe even after medication. Unable to speak in sentences.	EMS
	Yes, child is straining to breathe but not as severely as above. Not responding to usual inhaler medication. If child is not having trouble breathing, go to question 8.	2
4. Do you have a peak flow meter? How does the flow compare with the child's personal best?	Child's peak flow less than 50% of personal best.	2
5. Has the child been hospitalized or seen in the emergency room for asthma in the past year?	Yes.	2
6. Has steroid medication (such as prednisone [Prelone]) been prescribed for the child in the past year?	Yes.	2
7. How long has the child been coughing?	At least 2 to 3 days.	8
8. Describe the child's breathing (in child with previously diagnosed asthma).	No breathing difficulty but persistent mild cough.	8
9. Describe the child's symptoms (in a child not previously diagnosed with asthma).	Child has a cold and it sounds as if there may be wheezing.	8

EMS	= Activate EMS SYSTEM	**24-72**	= Appointment within 3 days
2	= See ASAP (within 1–2 hours)	**72+**	= Appointment in 4 days or more
8	= See same day		

High priority items appear in color.

51

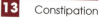
- Mineral oil can be an effective lubricant for chronic constipation. Its taste can be disguised in grape juice or chocolate milk. It should not be given to children who have a swallowing or vomiting disorder (for example, gastroesophageal reflux), in which aspiration is a risk. Children between 6 and 12 years of age should take 1 teaspoon to 1 tablespoon at bedtime; those over 12 should take 1 to 3 tablespoons.
- Osmotic preparations such as milk of magnesia increase the stool's water content. They are effective and generally safe. They should be taken at bedtime, followed by a 6- to 8-ounce glass of water. An appropriate dose of milk of magnesia is:
  - 2 to 5 years: 1–3 teaspoons
  - 6 to 11 years: 1–2 tablespoons
  - 12 or older: 2–4 tablespoons

Avoid stimulant laxatives such as phenolphthalein (Ex-Lax), bisacodyl (Dulcolax), or Senokot for children unless prescribed by the clinician.

In urgent situations in which rectal pain and impacted stool do not respond to other treatment, the clinician may recommend using a suppository or enema. If needed, glycerin suppositories provide gentle stimulation and rectal distention to promote a bowel movement. Dulcolax suppositories (10 mg bisacodyl) can be inserted as a full suppository for children over 12 years or use ˝ suppository for children between 6 and 12 years. This is usually prescribed as a one-time treatment.

To administer a suppository, if prescribed, have the child lie on one side. The suppository should be inserted pointed-end-first and pushed high into the rectum so it will not slip out. It should be retained for 15 to 20 minutes. If the suppository feels soft before you unwrap it, hold it under cold water for 1 to 2 minutes before unwrapping and inserting it. You may want to coat the tip with petroleum jelly (Vaseline) for easier insertion, especially if the child has an anal fissure.

If prescribed by the clinician, an enema can provide immediate relief of fecal impaction and rectal pain with the inability to pass stool. Sodium phosphate (Fleet Enema) comes in a squeeze bottle; mineral oil is also available. Use a children's size enema (2.25 ounces) for children between 4 and 12 years of age and an adult size (4.5 ounces) for those over 12. To administer the enema, have the child lie on his or her left side with the right knee bent. Remove the protective shield from the bottle and gently insert the enema tip into the rectum with the tip pointing toward the navel. Do not force the tip; use a slight side-to-side motion and wait for the muscles around the anus to relax. When in place, squeeze the bottle until nearly all the liquid is gone. Then have child sit on the toilet, but encourage him or her to try to resist evacuation for up to 5 minutes if possible.

CHAPTER 14

■ ■ ■ ■ ■ ■ ■ ■ ■ ■ ■ ■
■
■
■
■
■

Croup

Croup is a respiratory disorder characterized by a cough that sounds like a barking seal or a foghorn. It is also accompanied by noisy breathing (stridor), primarily during inspiration. Stridor is caused by a narrowed upper airway at the level of the larynx (voice box) and trachea. In contrast, lower airway obstruction results in wheezing or difficulty during expiration, as in asthma. There are four types of croup: viral croup, epiglottitis, spasmodic croup, and foreign body croup.

Viral croup is the most common form and occurs primarily in children between 6 months and 4 years of age. After several days of cold symptoms, the child develops a barky cough, noisy breathing, and in severe cases, respiratory distress. Fever is usually mild and the child does not appear ill. When the lower airway is also involved, wheezing may accompany the croup. More severe airway narrowing leads to retractions of the chest wall during respirations.

Epiglottitis is a serious bacterial infection and generally affects older children between the ages of 3 and 7 years. It is rapidly progressive and life threatening. The onset is usually abrupt, with drooling, high fever, sore throat, and strained breathing. The voice may sound muffled, and the child appears anxious and very ill.

Spasmodic (midnight) croup can affect any age group and recurrences are common. Onset is sudden, usually at night. It rarely progresses to airway obstruction. Other symptoms are absent and the child appears well between episodes.

Foreign body croup is rare but should always be suspected if the barky cough follows a choking episode, such as on a peanut or piece of a plastic toy.

> Mist inhalation is very effective in reducing the swelling of the upper airway. Humidifying the bedroom with a vaporizer or sitting in a steamy bathroom with the child cuddled in the parent's arms is the mainstay of treatment. Vomiting may give dramatic relief. Antibiotics are not indicated unless there is secondary bacterial infection such as otitis media. Cold medicines are not effective and may actually make the croup worse by excessively drying secretions. Parents should check the child frequently. The barking cough will persist, but if strained breathing develops or worsens, an office or emergency room visit is indicated. A parent should sleep in the same room with the child for close observation.

CROUP

Question	To See Clinician If . . .	When
1. Patient's name, telephone number, age		
2. Does cough sound like a barking seal? If so, how long has it been present?	Yes, present longer than 3 days.	2
3. Do the child's lips or skin look bluish?	Yes.	EMS
4. Is the child drooling or having difficulty swallowing?	Yes.	EMS
5. Has the child choked on something that could have stuck in the throat?	Yes.	EMS
6. Does the child make a loud noise when breathing?	Yes.	2
7. Is the child's chest caving in when breathing?	Yes.	2
8. Are there any other symptoms?	Earache, sore throat, fever above 101°F, or child looks ill.	2
9. Is the child lethargic or not drinking fluids well?	Yes.	2
10. Does the child have any other serious or chronic illness?	Diabetes, asthma, any kidney, respiratory, or heart disease.	2

EMS	= Activate EMS SYSTEM	24-72	= Appointment within 3 days
2	= See ASAP (within 1–2 hours)	72+	= Appointment in 4 days or more
8	= See same day		

High priority items appear in color.

ADVICE

If the child is playful, alert, and drinking fluids well, and if the croup is mild with no respiratory difficulty, home management is appropriate provided that the child will be observed closely. Callers should be given this advice:

- It is very important to relieve your child's anxiety by calm reassurance.
- Steam up the bathroom by running hot water from the shower. Close the door and sit in the thick steam with your child held on your lap for about 10 to 15 minutes. Repeat this three or four times during the day.
- Use a cool mist vaporizer in the child's bedroom. No medication needs to be added to the water. Run the vaporizer continuously.
- Do not give cold medications such as Sudafed or Benadryl, which could make the child worse. Acetaminophen (Tylenol) or ibuprofen can be given for fever.
- Call back immediately if any of the symptoms worsen or if the child's anxiety increases.

An appointment should automatically be given (ASAP: 1 to 2 hours) if the parents are distraught or have been up all night or if this is a second call for the same symptoms.

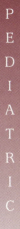

CHAPTER 15

■■■■■■■■■■■■
■
■
■
■

Diarrhea

Diarrhea is defined as an abnormal increase in either the number or water content of bowel movements. There are many causes of diarrhea. If the diarrhea is chronic (lasting longer than 1 week), an appointment is needed for an evaluation in the office. More commonly, the complaint is of the recent onset of acute symptoms. The cause of acute diarrhea is most often a viral infection of the intestinal tract (gastroenteritis). In young infants, diarrhea can also develop because of food intolerance (milk protein allergy; lactose or milk sugar intolerance). In addition, loose stools are frequently associated with upper respiratory illness, especially ear infections. Diarrhea caused by infection with intestinal viruses usually disappears within several days. Patients with marked diarrhea and mucus or blood in the stool, or diarrhea associated with high fever, should be given an appointment, because a bacterial organism may be identified. Prolonged diarrhea, with or without abdominal pain, can also be caused by parasites, such as Giardia from contaminated streams or water supply. After the initial intestinal infection is over, secondary lactose (milk sugar) intolerance can slow the recovery rate. Treatment for diarrhea is aimed at preventing dehydration (Table 15–1) by providing adequate fluid intake, and resting the bowel by avoiding solid foods.

For uncomplicated diarrhea, the following management is suggested:

1. All solid food, as well as milk and milk products, should be withheld for approximately 24 to 48 hours if diarrhea is severe.
2. During this period, fluid intake should be liberal. A special glucose-electrolyte solution called Pedialyte can be prescribed for infants. Older children can be given water, weak sweet tea, non-red Jell-O water, popsicles, or flat soft drinks (such as ginger ale, cola, or 7-Up), as well as Pedialyte. Fluids should be offered every 2 to 3 hours. Older children also may have pretzels, soda crackers, or dry toast, if desired.
3. For infants and younger children, on the second day, half-strength milk or half-strength formula may be started with gradually increasing small amounts of bland solid food, such as applesauce, lamb, boiled chicken, rice cereal, and boiled rice.
4. On the third day, full-strength milk or formula and a regular diet can be resumed provided the diarrhea has responded well (a decrease in number and in volume

TABLE 15–1 **Signs of Dehydration**
Listlessness
Dry tongue and inner cheek
Tears absent when crying
Sunken eyeballs
No urine in last 8–10 hours

of stools). If diarrhea persists, a trial of Isomil or ProSobee can be prescribed to eliminate lactose (milk sugar) from the diet.

5. For breastfed infants, breastfeeding should be continued. If the diarrhea is severe, offer Pedialyte in addition. If supplemental formula or other foods are being given, discontinue them for 12 to 24 hours.

Medications such as Kaopectate, paregoric, or Lomotil have no place in the routine treatment of diarrhea in children. They do not alter the course of the illness and can be quite harmful because they may mask the amount of fluid loss into the bowel and cause serious side effects.

DIARRHEA

Question	To See Clinician If . . .	When
1. Patient's name, telephone number, age	Per clinician preference.	
2. How many diarrheal stools have there been?	In an infant, more than 5 to 6 large, watery stools within 12 hours.	2
3. When did the child last urinate? Is his/her mouth moist? Other signs of dehydration? (See Advice)	Dehydration suspected.	2
4. Is there blood or mucus in the stool?	Yes, if either.	2
5. Does the child look unusually ill?	Yes.	2
6. Is there vomiting or abdominal pain?	Yes (either one).	2
7. Does the child have other symptoms?		
• Fever?	Over 103°F.	2
• Breathing fast and hard?	Yes.	2
• Jack-knifing knees to chest with severe cramps?	Yes.	2
• Earache?	Yes.	2
8. How long has diarrhea been present?	Longer than 7 days.	8
9. What is the usual state of the child's health?	Serious or chronic disease (e.g., diabetes).	8
10. Has the child been on a clear liquid diet? Has the diarrhea improved?	On clear liquid diet but diarrhea not responding after 24 hours.	8

SEE ALSO CHAPTER 28, VOMITING, OR CHAPTER 18, FEVER, IF APPROPRIATE.

EMS = Activate EMS SYSTEM	24-72 = Appointment within 3 days	
2 = See ASAP (within 1–2 hours)	72+ = Appointment in 4 days or more	
8 = See same day		

High priority items appear in color.

ADVICE

If the child is alert, active, and does not appear unusually ill, and if diarrhea is mild and infrequent (less than six stools in the past 12 hours without blood or mucus), feeding advice and home management are appropriate. The parent should be advised to watch for signs of dehydration (see Table 15–1) and call back if it is suspected. The major objective of treatment is to prevent dehydration by providing fluids to replace what is lost in the diarrhea.

Review of Diet

- Clear liquids: water, Jell-O water, weak sweet tea, or flat soft drinks (flat to avoid gas) for 24 hours or until diarrhea subsides. (To make Jell-O water, dissolve a regular-size package of powder in 1 cup of hot water, then add 4 more cups of cool water. Avoid red-colored flavors, which can be confused with blood.) Offer such liquids every 2 hours. Pedialyte can be used for infants, or Pedialyte popsicles for older children.
- As diarrhea subsides, on the second to third days, infants can progress to the BRAT diet (**b**anana, dry **r**ice cereal mixed with water, **a**pplesauce, and dry **t**oast).
- If child is under the age of 1 year, diluted Isomil (formula containing no milk sugar) can be started after clear liquids (¼ strength on first day, ½ strength on second day, and then full strength). Continue full strength for 5 days and then resume normal formula or milk.
- Breastfed infants should continue breastfeeding but should not receive supplemental formula or other foods. They may be given Pedialyte as a supplement if the diarrhea is severe.

Other Care

- If a diaper rash appears, expose the skin to air and then use a thick coat of petroleum jelly (Vaseline) to protect the skin.
- If fever is present, see Chapter 18.
- If the child is vomiting, see Chapter 28.

CHAPTER 16

■ ■ ■ ■ ■ ■ ■ ■ ■ ■ ■ ■ ■ ■

Earache

There are basically three types of ear infections, two affecting the middle ear and one affecting the outer ear:

- Acute otitis media (AOM): bacterial infection of the middle ear
- Otitis media with effusion (OME): fluid in the middle ear, sometimes associated with bacterial infection, but also associated with other causes
- Otitis externa: external ear infection, also known as "swimmer's ear"

Acute Otitis Media

This kind of marked ear pain or throbbing usually begins 2 to 3 days after an uncomplicated cold. Less commonly, the onset is abrupt and unexpected. AOM is often associated with irritability and fever. Infants and young children unable to verbalize their complaints frequently tug at their ear. The pain may awaken the child from sleep. Occasionally a child will have decreased hearing or disturbed balance.

A discharge of pus or blood from the ear signifies rupture of the eardrum (tympanic membrane). This sometimes causes an associated external canal infection.

Treatment of otitis media is aimed at minimizing pain and discomfort, treating the infection with specific antibiotic therapy, and returning the ear to normal function by reopening the eustachian tube (the tubelike structure that connects the middle ear to the area behind the nose) if it is blocked. If antibiotic treatment is prescribed, it must be continued for the full 10-day course of therapy.

> Maximal compliance with the treatment plan is essential and should be reinforced by instructions whenever possible. That is, parents must be told specifically to continue use of antibiotics for the entire prescribed duration and frequency, rather than stopping when the pain is gone.

Otitis Media with Effusion

OME is characterized by fleeting ear pain or discomfort, "popping," or a feeling of stuffiness in the affected ear. Decreased hearing and, to a lesser extent, disturbed balance are common. The incidence of OME is higher in allergic patients. Fluid in the middle ear without infection may follow AOM. Often fluid persists for 1 to 3 months after AOM and then resolves spontaneously without adverse consequences. If OME persists longer than 3 months, consultation with an ear, nose, and throat (ENT) specialist may be considered.

As already mentioned, one of the aims of therapy for otitis media is to reopen the eustachian tube, allowing aeration and drainage from the middle ear. If OME persists longer than 3 months or hearing loss occurs, tubes in the middle ear may be recommended.

CHAP

Eye
Infla

Conjunctivi

Conjunctivitis, (
white of the eye
(mechanical or c

Bacterial Conju

Bacterial conjunc
lids, with intense
eral weeks if untr
nosis and to rule
effective treatme
while using topic
change to a more
infection, separat
child is considere
gone for 24 hours

Viral Conjunctiv

Viral conjunctiviti
purulent discharg
ary bacterial infe
viral conjunctiviti
ments for an exar

Allergic Conjun

In spring and fal
swelling, and a w.
or asthma. The co
presses afford son
tihistamines. Beca
are best seen. An
diagnosed, the pa
seasons.

Otitis Externa

Otitis externa, or "swimmer's ear," is an infection of the skin that lines the ear's outer canal, commonly associated with swimming in pools and, less commonly, in the ocean or lakes. It can also result when the eardrum ruptures during an episode of acute otitis media and discharges pus and bacteria into the canal. The presence of moisture and swimming pool chemicals in the ear canal softens the skin and provides a favorable environment for infection. Pain is occasionally severe, and there may be fever.

A hallmark of otitis externa is marked pain when the outer ear is moved or touched, a situation not observed in the more common middle ear infection.

Most cases of otitis externa will respond to antibiotic-cortisone (Cortisporin Otic) eardrops used four times daily for 7 to 10 days. Pain is relieved by acetaminophen (Tylenol) or ibuprofen (Motrin) and gentle heat applied over the outer ear using a heating pad or hot water bottle. As for otitis media, it is important that instructions be followed carefully, because this usually mild disease may worsen and cause severe pain if treatment is incomplete. If improvement is not seen within 36 to 48 hours, or if symptoms become worse, the child should be seen for further evaluation.

Is High Fever Harmful?

Contrary to popular belief, fever is rarely dangerous or harmful to the brain, even at levels of 104°F lasting for several days. In fact, fever is a sign that the body's defense mechanism is working properly. In the 1- to 5-year age group, fever may precipitate a convulsion, but it is more likely that the rate of rise rather than the actual height of fever sets off the seizure. A febrile seizure usually occurs very early in the course of the illness and often precedes the awareness that fever is present. Temperature greater than 105°F, however, is associated with a greater risk of serious bacterial infection such as meningitis or sepsis.

Management of Fever

Infants and children can be kept comfortable with appropriate doses of antifever medication while being observed at home or after the nature of the illness has been defined by the clinician. Side effects of the medication are minimized by prescribing the correct dose of either acetaminophen-containing drugs (Tylenol, Tempra) (Table 18–1) or a nonsteroidal anti-inflammatory drug (NSAID) such as ibuprofen (e.g., Motrin or Advil) (Table 18–2).

> Fever is a healthy sign that the body is responding to infection and is not by itself harmful. Treating the fever does not treat the illness; the objective of treatment is to keep the child comfortable and reduce the possibility of a fever convulsion in children 1 to 5 years old.

Infants younger than 3 months should be seen in the office for any temperature over 100.4°F rectally because they are difficult to evaluate without an examination. The same is true for infants between 3 and 6 months who have rectal temperatures greater than 101°F.

TELEPHO

EARACI

Question

1. Patient's n
   number, a

2. How sever

3. Has the pa
   sleep?

4. How have

5. Is there a d
   from the ea

6. Does the ch

7. How long h

8. Does the ch
   swimming?
   hurt when it

EMS = Activ

2 = See /

8 = See s

A D V I C

Parents shou

- If the pain
  should be
- Apply gent
  Sometimes
  20 minutes
- If pain occi
  vide relief.
- If the eardi
  should sche
- For swimm
  Pull the ear
  plug placed
- Children wi
- If necessar
  pain medic.

TABLE 18-1 Managing Fever with Acetaminophen*: Doses Every 4–6 Hours

Age	Weight	Oral Drops (Full Dropper = 80 mg, 0.8 mL)	Liquid 160 mg/tsp (5 mL)	Baby Chewable Tablets (80 mg)	Junior Chewable Tablets or Caplets (160 mg)	Adult Tablets or Caplets (325 mg)
0–3 months	6–11 lb (2.5–5.4 kg)	½ dropper (0.4 mL)				
4–11 months	12–17 lb (5.5–7.9 kg)	1 dropper (0.8 mL)	½ tsp			
12–23 months	18–23 lb (8.0–10.9 kg)	1½ dropper (1.2 mL)	¾ tsp			
2–3 years	24–35 lb (11.0–15.9 kg)	2 droppers (1.6 mL)	1 tsp	2 tablets		
4–5 years	36–47 lb (16.0–21.9 kg)		1½ tsp	3 tablets		
6–8 years	48–59 lb (22.0–26.9 kg)		2 tsp	4 tablets	2 tablets or caplets	
9–10 years	60–71 lb (27.0–31.9 kg)		2½ tsp	5 tablets	2½ tablets or caplets	
11 years	72–95 lb (32.0–43.9 kg)		3 tsp	6 tablets	3 tablets or caplets	
12 years and over	96 lb (44.0 kg) or more				4 tablets or caplets	1 or 2 tablets or caplets

*Tylenol, Tempra, Panodol, Liquiprin. The acetaminophen dose ranges from 10–15 mg/kg (5–7.5 mg/lb).

TABLE 18–2 Managing Fever with Children's Ibuprofen*: Doses Every 6–8 Hours

Age	Weight	Pediatric Drops 50 mg per 1.25 mL (1 dropper)	Suspension 100 mg per 5 mL (1 teaspoon)	Chewable Tablets (50 mg per tablet)	Chewable Tablets (100 mg per tablet)	Swallowable Caplets (100 mg per caplet)
0–5 months	Under 12 lb (5.4 kg)	Do not use	Do not use			
6–11 months	12–17 lb (5.5–7.9 kg)	½ dropper	½ tsp			
12–23 months	18–23 lb (8.0–10.9 kg)	1½ to 2 droppers	¾ to 1 tsp			
2–3 years	24–35 lb (11.0–15.9 kg)	2 droppers	1 tsp	2 tablets		
4–5 years	36–47 lb (16.0–21.9 kg)		1½ tsp	3 tablets		
6–8 years	48–59 lb (22.0–26.9 kg)		2 tsp	4 tablets	2 tablets	2 caplets
9–10 years	60–71 lb (27.0–31.9 kg)		2½ tsp	5 tablets	2½ tablets	2 caplets
11 years	72–95 lb (32.0–43.9 kg)		3 tsp	6 tablets	3 tablets	3 caplets

*Advil, Motrin. These dosages should not be given more than four times a day. The ibuprofen dose ranges from 5–10 mg/kg (2.2–4.5 mg/lb). The recommended OTC dose is 7.5 mg/kg (3.4 mg/lb). The dose for maximum effect is 10 mg/kg (4.5 mg/lb).

FEVER

Question	To See Clinician If . . .	When
1. Patient's name, telephone number, age	Under age 3 months if temperature above 100.4°F rectally regardless of any other symptom	2
2. How is the child acting?	Appears unusually ill, irritable, or lethargic	2
3. Has the child ever had a convulsion?	Yes	2
4. How long has the fever been present? What is the actual temperature?	Fever present over 48 hours without explanation or any fever over 103°F rectally or orally	8
5. Are there any other symptoms?		
• Headache or stiff neck?	Stiff neck or headache out of proportion to fever	2
• Rapid or difficult breathing?	Yes	2
• Rash?	Small red or purplish spots (looking like blood spots or bruising under the skin) that do not go away with pressure (petechiae)	2
• Urinary burning or frequency? (Ask about amount and type of fluid intake)	Yes	2
• Ear, nose, or throat problems?	Cough, sneezing, sore throat, or earache	8
• Vomiting, diarrhea, or abdominal pain?	Yes	8
6. What is the child's usual state of health?	Any serious or chronic disorder, such as diabetes, cystic fibrosis, asthma, seizures, etc.	8

EMS = Activate EMS SYSTEM		24-72 = Appointment within 3 days	
2 = See ASAP (within 1–2 hours)		72+ = Appointment in 4 days or more	
8 = See same day			

High priority items appear in color.

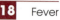
ADVICE

The child should be seen if there is any doubt about the seriousness of the illness. The illness may be treated by home management phone advice under the following conditions:

- If the child is playful or not acting particularly ill, fussy, or lethargic.
- If associated respiratory or gastrointestinal symptoms are mild and the telephone review of systems, question 5, is essentially negative.
- If illness in other family members with similar symptoms is very mild.
- If the parent feels comfortable with the home advice disposition.

The parent should always be instructed to call back if the symptoms worsen or change significantly.

General Management Recommendations

- Increase the child's intake of fluids (popsicles, juice, flat sodas, Jell-O, water).
- Give medicine regularly (every 4 to 6 hours for acetaminophen or every 6 to 8 hours for ibuprofen) until the fever is under 101°F or the child is comfortable.
- Both acetaminophen and ibuprofen are equally effective for most children. Do not give more than the recommended dose (see Tables 18–1 and 18–2 or follow the clinician's instructions). **Do not** use aspirin, which is associated with a rare disease, Reye's Syndrome.
- Acetaminophen preparations (e.g., Tylenol, Tempra) contain different concentrations. Always read the label carefully. The desired dosage is 5 to 7.5 mg per pound of body weight (maximum 600 mg at any one time for children).
- Ibuprofen preparations (Motrin, Advil) also come in different concentrations. The desired dosage for fever is 7.5 to 10 mg of over-the counter preparation per kg of body weight (3 to 5 mg per pound). The most common gastrointestinal side effects are nausea, heartburn, and possibly bleeding ulcers. Do not use ibuprofen if the child is less than 6 months old or is allergic to aspirin. Be cautious about using ibuprofen if the child is very dehydrated or has a history of asthma (hyperactive airway disease) or kidney problems.
- Dosage by weight is more accurate than by age.
- Do not leave medication within the reach of children, and always replace the cap immediately.
- Rectal thermometers (glass with short round bulb) and high-quality ear thermometers are the most accurate; digital thermometers can be used to take temperatures by rectum, mouth, or under the armpit (which registers approximately 1°F lower). In some places, glass thermometers containing mercury are being recalled because of the danger of toxicity if they are broken.

Sponging Instructions

Sponging is only an adjunct recommended for the temporary relief of symptoms when the fever is over 103°F. The principle is to promote heat loss via evaporation, similar to the cool feeling experienced when leaving a swimming pool.

- Use plain water at room temperature. Never use cold water, ice, or alcohol because these might cause shivering, which raises body temperature.
- Do not immerse the body in water or cover with wash cloths. This impedes evaporation. Use a partially filled tub.
- Rub a wet cloth or sponge briskly over the arms, legs, and trunk, and then let the water evaporate from the surface of the skin.
- Stop sponging immediately if shivering occurs.
- Sponge for only 15 to 20 minutes, one time. By then the medication will have begun to work.

CHAPTER 19

■ ■ ■ ■ ■ ■ ■ ■ ■ ■ ■ ■ ■

Headache

Headaches can be acute (of recent onset) or chronic and recurrent (long-standing). Most acute headaches are associated with infectious illnesses like colds, influenza, or sinusitis. Frequently, a fever itself causes a headache. One of the most serious infections associated with headache is meningitis, a bacterial or viral infection of the lining covering the brain and spinal canal. In meningitis, the child appears seriously ill, often has a stiff neck, and is extremely irritable. In encephalitis, a viral brain infection, the headache is often throbbing and associated with vomiting. Drowsiness and abnormal behavior are common.

> Whenever headache is accompanied by mental confusion, immediate medical care is urgently needed.

Chronic and recurring headaches are extremely common complaints among children. Perhaps the most common cause is stress and tension, reflecting the fast pace and lifestyle of today's families. The typical history of a tension headache is constant dull pain and pressure in the forehead and muscles at the base of the skull that occur more frequently at the end of the day. The diagnosis of tension headache is one of exclusion, because headaches can be caused by any number of more serious medical problems. These include childhood migraine, sinus infections, dental problems, high blood pressure (commonly described as throbbing), and brain tumors, in which the headache often awakens the child from sleep and is worse after lying down. It may be associated with early morning vomiting, which relieves the pain.

Because all patients with persisting or chronic headache need an examination, the role of the telephone assistant is to help decide upon the timing of the appointment. Any patient with an acute headache, or a patient who is acting ill or is in severe pain, needs to be seen right away. If the headache has been long-standing, if there has been no recent change in pattern, and if the child is in school and functioning normally, a future appointment is advisable. As with any problem, the earliest possible appointment should be arranged.

> If the level of parental anxiety is high, that alone should prompt an appointment as soon as possible.

TELEPHONE DECISION GUIDELINES

HEADACHE

Question	To See Clinician If . . .	When
1. Patient's name, telephone number, age		
2. Are there any associated symptoms, such as vomiting, stiff neck, difficulty with vision, recent change of behavior or personality, or drowsiness?	Yes.	2
3. How often do the headaches occur?	Daily.	2
4. Are the headaches getting worse or better?	Becoming more painful or more frequent.	2
5. Are you treating them with any medication? Does it help?	Headaches do not respond to treatment.	2
6. Has the child had a recent head injury?	Yes.	2
7. Is the child vomiting? Does vomiting occur in the early morning?	Yes.	2
8. Does the child seem anxious?	Yes.	2
9. Does the child have any other serious or chronic medical disorder, such as allergic rhinitis, diabetes, asthma, previous sinus infection?	Yes.	8
10. How long have the headaches been occurring?	More than a month (and child is not ill and has no associated symptoms).	24-72

EMS = Activate EMS SYSTEM	24-72 = Appointment within 3 days	
2 = See ASAP (within 1–2 hours)	72+ = Appointment in 4 days or more	
8 = See same day		

High priority items appear in color.

ADVICE

- For relief of headache, have the child lie down to rest and place a cold washcloth over the forehead.
- If the headache persists, give acetaminophen (Tylenol) or a nonsteroidal anti-inflammatory drug such as ibuprofen (Motrin, Advil).

CHAPTER 20

■ ■ ■ ■ ■ ■ ■ ■ ■ ■ ■ ■ ■ ■

Head Injury

The complaint of head injury is very common, one that few children escape. It is important for telephone triage staff to be aware that the clinician's role in evaluating children with head injury is to decide on the necessity for consultation with a neurosurgeon and hospitalization for either treatment or observation. Very few children require these measures, but a careful evaluation in the office and very close follow-up at home are essential elements of management.

Not all head injuries are concussions. Injury to the brain can occur in several ways, the concussion being the most common. A concussion is a form of closed head injury (that is, the skull is intact) in which there is a brief loss of consciousness, unusual behavior, or mental confusion followed by gradual recovery. Not all children with concussions lose consciousness. Sometimes the major symptoms of a concussion are temporary loss of vision, pallor, listlessness, memory loss, or vomiting. Symptoms may persist for many hours or pass quickly. Very few children require hospitalization. The exceptions are those with severe head injuries (causing mental confusion, for instance) or frank bleeding into the brain as with a subdural or epidural hematoma. The disturbed mental status in these extremely serious conditions is more profound, and there are neurologic deficits. Often the child has been in a serious accident and shows signs of multiple trauma to other parts of the body, such as fractures and internal abdominal injuries. These children must be hospitalized immediately.

The more common complaint for which most parents call the office is that their child has fallen and hit his or her head. If the fall was a significant one (for instance, from a tree), it is best to bring the child into the office for an examination. If the fall was trivial, however (such as from a bed or sofa onto a carpeted floor), and the child is acting fine, it is appropriate to explain what signs and symptoms should be watched for at home, with instructions to call back if there is a significant change. The most important factor in evaluating the effects of head injury is what happens to the child over time. Initially, mild symptoms such as pallor or a few episodes of vomiting are common; it is what develops after these initial symptoms that must be observed closely. Skull x-ray films are of little help in this regard. The presence of a skull fracture by itself usually will not influence management. Conversely, the absence of a skull fracture does not rule out the possibility of a serious brain injury. Close observation is essential in either case, and good parental supervision at home is critical.

A bump or bruise (contusion) on the head following an injury represents bleeding into the skin (hematoma). A bump or bruise on the forehead should be expected to change color from purple to yellow, and sometimes the discoloration will spread into the area around the eyes. The bruise usually resolves in about 7 to 10 days.

> If the history of trauma raises suspicions of child abuse, the child should be given an appointment as quickly as possible.

HEAD INJURY

Question	To See Clinician If . . .	When
1. Patient's name, telephone number, age		
2. When did the injury occur? Did the child lose consciousness or have a convulsion?	The child was unconscious for more than a few seconds or has had a convulsion.	EMS
3. Has the child had other symptoms: Mental confusion or strange behavior? Vomiting? Loss of vision? Pallor? Lethargy? Very brief loss of consciousness?	Yes, and abnormal behavior or confusion is continuing.	EMS
	Yes, but the child now appears to be acting normally.	2
4. Has any blood or fluid come from the child's nose or ears?	Yes.	2
5. Has the child had a fever or stiff neck since the injury?	Yes.	2
6. Does the child have a headache?	Yes.	2
7. Did you see the accident? How did it happen?	High fall (for example, from a tree), automobile accident, or strong blow or if description raises suspicion of child abuse.	2
8. Does the child show any evidence of another injury, such as a cut, scrape, abdominal pain, or failure to use an arm or leg?	Yes.	2
9. Has the child had a head injury in the past?	Yes.	8

EMS = Activate EMS SYSTEM	24-72	= Appointment within 3 days
2 = See ASAP (within 1–2 hours)	72+	= Appointment in 4 days or more
8 = See same day		

High priority items appear in color.

ADVICE

If the caller did not witness the injury, ask if anyone else saw it, such as a teacher. Any witness should be asked for as detailed a description as possible.

If the child is acting normally and shows no symptoms of concussion, and if the injury was slight, the child can be observed at home for any of the following:

- Severe or increasing headache
- Persistent vomiting (for example, more than three times)
- Dizziness or unsteadiness when walking
- Excessive or persistent drowsiness
- Slurred speech
- Clear or bloody discharge from nose or ears
- Unequal size of the pupils (the black part of the eye)

The child may be sleepy after the injury. Allow a nap but awaken the child in 1 hour to reevaluate and to make sure behavior is normal.

Acetaminophen (Tylenol) or ibuprofen (Motrin, Advil) can be used for relief of headache or for the local pain of a bruise.

During that night, the child should be awakened at midnight, 3 A.M., and 6 A.M. to make sure he or she is arousable and acts normal.

CHAPTER 21

. . . .

Insect Bites and Stings

Insect bites and children go together, and concerns about Lyme disease, itchy mosquito bites, and bee stings announce that summer is here. The bite or sting of an insect can be painful because of reactions to the chemical material injected into the skin, but usually it is not dangerous. Symptoms can be local (confined to the area of the bite) or generalized (spreading to other parts of the body). Generalized reactions are potentially dangerous because of an overwhelming allergic reaction leading to shock (anaphylaxis). Although this type of reaction is rare, the potential danger of an insect bite should always be kept in mind.

Local Reactions

Most insect bites and stings of hymenoptera (wasps, bees, hornets, and yellow jackets) are not serious and usually require no special care. If the stinger can be seen, it should be extracted by scraping it off with a knife blade or a fingernail. There may be marked local swelling that occasionally involves an entire hand or foot. Itching, burning, and stinging are common responses to a bite. Pressure with an ice cube may relieve the pain and swelling. Topical application of calamine lotion or an antihistamine taken by mouth can be used for further relief.

Generalized Reaction

A generalized reaction can include a dry cough, a sense of chest or throat constriction, swelling or itching around the eyes, hives, wheezing, pallor, and a sense of anxiety.

> Serious allergic symptoms may occur within the first few minutes following the sting. In some cases, symptoms may progress to life-threatening shock (called anaphylaxis) requiring immediate emergency treatment with activation of the EMS or 911 system.

Once it has been determined that a patient is susceptible to a generalized rather than local reaction, prevention of future bites is of prime importance. Warm weather heralds the peak of sting season. Careful inspection of home and grounds should be made to detect and carefully eliminate nests during the summer, when insects are naturally more aggressive. Perfumes, hairspray, and scented skin lotions should be avoided. Going barefoot invites problems. Insect repellents such as Off may be used on outings. Following a generalized reaction, a program of desensitization or "allergy shots" should be considered in consultation with an allergist. Such shots should not be depended upon to totally prevent a serious reaction, however. For this reason, a bee sting emergency kit (e.g., EpiPen) is prescribed to keep at home. Proper instructions must be given in its use, and the EpiPen should always accompany the patient on outings.

INSECT BITES AND STINGS

Question	To See Clinician If . . .	When
1. Patient's name, telephone number, age		
2. Is the child having any difficulty breathing? Lightheadedness? Swelling around the eyes? Widespread rash all over the body? Difficulty swallowing? Tingling or sensation of a thickened tongue?	Yes. (An EpiPen injection should be given while waiting for EMS to arrive, if it is available and the caller has been instructed in its use.)	EMS
3. Did you see what bit the child?	Spider, scorpion, or centipede.	2
4. Has the child had a serious local allergic reaction to an insect bite before?	Yes.	2
5. How long ago was the bite? If more than 24 hours, is the area getting redder or more swollen?	Yes.	2
6. Is the child acting ill?	Yes.	2
7. If the child was bitten by a tick more than 24 hours ago, is there any fever, headache, rash, or muscle aches?	Yes.	2
8. If the insect was a tick, is the tick embedded in the skin?	Yes. See tick removal advice in Advice box. Appointment needed if tick removal is not successful.	8
9. Is the area around the bite red, very swollen, or itchy? Has ice been applied? Was an antihistamine given? (e.g., Benadryl, Chlor-Trimeton)	Yes, and ice and antihistamine did not help.	8
10. Does the bite look infected?	Yes.	8

EMS = Activate EMS SYSTEM	**24-72** = Appointment within 3 days	
2 = See ASAP (within 1–2 hours)	**72+** = Appointment in 4 days or more	
8 = See same day		

High priority items appear in color.

ADVICE

- Cold compresses or ice can be applied to reduce the swelling. If the bite is very itchy, an antihistamine such as Benadryl or Chlor-Trimeton can be given by mouth.
- If there are generalized symptoms (such as difficulty breathing or swallowing, or feeling faint) an emergency EpiPen kit should be used if one is available in the home and the caller was previously instructed in its use. The child should also take an antihistamine right away. Call 911 without delay. Do not bother with any managed-care authorization requirements on hospital or emergency room use. Keep the patient on the line.

Tick Removal Advice

- Cover the tick with nail polish remover or alcohol.
- Grasp the body of the tick firmly with tweezers and remove the head from the child's skin by pulling slowly, steadily, and gently.
- Do **not** use a match or cigarette.

CHAPTER 22

▪ ▪ ▪ ▪ ▪ ▪ ▪ ▪ ▪ ▪ ▪ ▪

Nosebleed

Nosebleeds (epistaxis) are common in young children. Although the experience can be frightening, particularly because it often occurs at night, a nosebleed rarely causes severe blood loss.

The telephone assessment of nosebleed in a child has four purposes:

- To instruct parents in the proper way to stop the bleeding.
- To eliminate suspicions of a serious underlying bleeding disorder, such as thrombocytopenic (low platelets) purpura, leukemia, or hemophilia, by asking a few simple questions about the child's history and family history of bleeding problems. Fortunately, these bleeding disorders are very rare.
- To instruct parents in prevention and to alert them to the possibility that chronic blood loss from repeated small bleeds over a long period may result in anemia (as shown by pallor or fatigue).
- To advise when to call back if the initial decision is that the problem can be managed at home.

The lining of the septum of the nose contains many tiny blood vessels. Because of local irritation from dryness or from sneezing caused by a cold or allergy, these tiny vessels may break and bleed. Foreign bodies in the nose also can cause bleeding, often with an associated foul-smelling discharge of pus. Nosebleeds commonly follow injury, nose blowing or picking, and nasal infections.

> Most nosebleeds can be stopped by firm pressure produced by pinching the nostrils closed for a full 5 minutes without letting up or peeking to see if it has stopped. The child should be placed in a sitting position, **not** lying down or with the head tilted backward.

Parents should try to remain calm and reassure the child, because apprehension will make treatment more difficult. If bleeding restarts, the nose pinching pressure should be reapplied for a longer period of time (10 minutes) with a pledget of cotton coated with petroleum jelly placed in the nostril.

Rarely, a child may have difficulty with blood clotting. The parent should be asked if anyone else in the family has a clotting problem, if the child also has bleeding from other sites (such as the gums), or if the child has more than the usual number of bruises. If there is no family history of a bleeding disorder and the child has no other history of bleeding, a clotting disorder is virtually ruled out if the nosebleed ceases with conventional treatment. Occasionally, nosebleeds are associated with high blood pressure.

If the bleeding does not stop after adequate home management, or if there are multiple recurrences, the child should be evaluated in the office for possible cauterization of the blood vessels in the nose. If there is a specific underlying predisposing factor, like allergic rhinitis or dryness secondary to lack of humidity in the home, treatment of that problem should help prevent further nosebleeds. If the nose is very dry, a small amount of petroleum jelly (Vaseline) applied by Q-tip just inside the nostril may help. The child's use of aspirin, ibuprofen (Motrin, Advil), or other nonsteroidal anti-inflammatory drugs, which can interfere with blood clotting, should be limited.

NOSEBLEED

Question	To See Clinician If . . .	When
1. Patient's name, telephone number, age		
2. Is the nose bleeding now? How long has it been bleeding?	Yes, has been bleeding for more than 30 minutes and parent is unable to stop it.	EMS
3. Was the nose injured?	Yes.	2
4. Is there bleeding from any other source (gums, urine, bowel movement, bruises)?	Yes.	2
5. Does anyone else in the family have difficulty with clotting?	Yes.	2
6. Has the child had other nosebleeds recently?	More than three bleeds in the past 48 hours. Several in the past few months.	2 / 24-72
7. Does the child have any other symptoms?	Dizzy, fever greater than 101°F, looks pale or ill.	2
8. Does the child have any serious or chronic medical problem?	Diabetes; asthma; kidney, respiratory, or heart disease.	8

EMS = Activate EMS SYSTEM		**24-72** = Appointment within 3 days
2 = See ASAP (within 1–2 hours)		**72+** = Appointment in 4 days or more
8 = See same day		

High priority items appear in color.

ADVICE

Give advice to stop bleeding:

- Place the child in a sitting position, **not** lying down. Do not tilt the head backward (may cause blood to run down the throat).
- Soak a washcloth in ice water and use it to pinch the nostrils closed for a full 5 minutes without letting go.
- If bleeding recurs, repeat. Coat a small wad of cotton with petroleum jelly (Vaseline), place it in the affected nostril, and pinch the nostrils shut for a full 10 minutes. Most nosebleeds will stop with 10 to 30 minutes of direct pressure.
- Each night for 1 week, apply a small amount of petroleum jelly just inside each nostril to prevent crust formation.
- If the heat is on in the house, humidify the child's bedroom to prevent reoccurrence due to dryness.

  If the child's nose has been injured, the child should be examined to rule out the possibility of a fracture.

CHAPTER 23

■ ■ ■ ■ ■ ■ ■ ■ ■ ■ ■ ■ ■ ■

Poisoning

Accidental poisonings of children are a major, year-round concern. Accidents and poisonings in the United States account for the largest number of deaths among children—more than the next seven causes of fatalities combined. Children are by nature curious and love to experiment. The following features of accidental childhood poisoning suggest the kinds of precautions that may help:

- Two-thirds of all cases reported involve children under 5 years of age.
- Most of these ingestions occur in the presence of an adult and in the late afternoon, when the product is in use and the childproof cap is off.
- The most hazardous location for accidental poisoning in the home is the kitchen. (Look beneath the sink.)
- Acetaminophen (Tylenol, Tempra, Liquiprin), household detergents and bleach, plants, cough and cold preparations, and vitamins lead the list of poisons. Tranquilizer poisoning is on the increase.
- Other frequently ingested substances are drain cleaners (such as Drano and Liquid-Plumr), turpentine, kerosene, furniture polish, paints, and many other household preparations.
- Aspirin—a declining cause of accidental childhood poisoning in the United States—can, in large doses, cause deep, rapid breathing, dehydration, fever, increased acidity of the blood (acidosis), convulsions, coma, and death.
- Ingestion of vitamin preparations that contain iron (primarily adult formulations of prenatal iron-containing products) can cause vomiting of blood, diarrhea, liver inflammation (hepatitis), coma, shock, and death.

Simple steps to "poison-proof" the home can go far in eliminating accidental ingestion of poisons by children:

- All household products and medications **must** be kept out of sight and reach of children and should be kept in a locked cabinet or closet. When adults are using a medication, they must be careful to keep it out of the reach of small children.

Two-thirds of poisonings from household medications occur because the medicine was not returned to its usual storage place. Also, a medicine chest filled with half-empty leftover bottles is dangerous. Medicine cabinets should be cleaned out periodically. The safest way to dispose of unused medicines, both liquids and pills, is to flush them down the toilet. Bottles that contained liquid medicine should be rinsed with water before they are tossed in the wastebasket.

- Medicine should be called "medicine"—not "candy." Candy-flavored medications and vitamins present the greatest temptation.
- Medications should be kept apart from other household products and in their original, properly labeled containers. **Always check the label and dosage before administering a medication.**

- When storing household products such as bleaches, polishes, and insecticides, avoid the use of easily accessible cabinets.
- Request the safest child-resistant medicine containers whenever possible.

If, despite all precautions, a child does ingest a medication or another household substance, parents should call their physician or the local poison control center for advice on the potential danger and need for further therapy. If a parent calls the office and you are uncertain, tell the parent you will put them on hold while you call the poison control center for information.

When a parent is advised to bring a child who has ingested a substance to the office, they should be instructed to bring the original container so that the ingredients can be verified.

Syrup of Ipecac

Parents can be instructed to administer ipecac syrup to their child. Ipecac syrup is a reliable emetic—that is, a substance that induces vomiting. **It should be given only on instruction from a physician or poison control center.** Two teaspoons can be safely administered to infants 9 to 12 months old, after the child drinks about 4 ounces of warm water. The dosage for a child 1 to 4 years of age is 3 teaspoonfuls (1 tablespoon) given after drinking 4 to 8 ounces of warm water. Vomiting will usually occur within 15 or 20 minutes after the administration of the ipecac.

Vomiting should never be induced after the ingestion of lye, petroleum products, or other corrosive substances; in infants younger than 9 months; or in children who are stuporous or who have ingested substances that are likely to make them stuporous or unconscious, because of the risk of aspiration (inhaling vomitus into the lungs).

Although it is advantageous for all families with children younger than 5 years to have syrup of ipecac in the home, they should remember that **it is to be administered only on instruction from a physician or poison control center and should be safely locked up.**

POISONING

Question	To See Clinician If . . .	When
1. Patient's name, telephone number, age		
2. What is patient's status? (alert, drowsy?)	Lethargic, drowsy, confused, hyperirritable, obvious lesions such as mouth or skin burns, or any symptoms resulting from ingestion, such as vomiting or abdominal pain.	EMS
3. How much time has elapsed since ingestion?	If child is acting mentally normal and • Time of ingestion is unknown. • Time of ingestion is more than 4 hours ago.	2
4. What is nature of substance ingested? (Trade and/or generic name)	All corrosives (strong acids, alkalis such as lye). ***Do not induce vomiting.***	EMS
	Hydrocarbons (kerosene, paint thinners, turpentine, furniture polish). ***Do not induce vomiting.***	EMS
	All insecticides, rodenticides (rat poisons).	EMS
	All narcotics and tranquilizers (methadone, tricyclics such as imipramine, amitriptyline—Tofranil, Elavil), or ***any*** unknown pills.	EMS
	Most other pills (e.g., iron, vitamins, sleeping medications, barbiturates, aspirin). Note: Some pills (antihistamines, compazine, barbiturates) will have antivomiting effects, making syrup of ipecac less effective.	2
	All plants, seeds, berries, wild mushrooms.	2
5. Has vomiting already taken place?	Yes, and substance ingested was a corrosive or a petroleum distillate. Yes, but substance ingested was nontoxic: Home management is appropriate.	EMS
6. What information is available on the label of the ingested substance (antidotes, first aid, etc.)?	Substance extremely toxic Substance potentially toxic Substance nontoxic Unsure about toxicity	EMS 2 Home management Call Poison Control Center

POISONING (Continued)

Question	To See Clinician If . . .	When
7. Has poison control been called?	Poison Control Center (PCC) so advises (based on potential toxicity)	Per PCC instruction

EMS = Activate EMS SYSTEM	**24-72** = Appointment within 3 days
2 = See ASAP (within 1–2 hours)	**72+** = Appointment in 4 days or more
8 = See same day	

High priority items appear in color.

ADVICE

Be sure you obtain the patient's name, address, and phone number. Many parents will neglect to provide them in their haste and panic. If possible, you should also record what the substance was, how much was ingested, the age and weight of the child, and whether syrup of ipecac is available.

Ingestions Requiring Medical Attention

- If the time of ingestion is unknown, do not take the time at home to induce vomiting (even if indicated). If the child is alert, follow immediate first aid measures at home, then bring the child immediately to the office. If the child is mentally confused or drowsy, it is safer to take the child to the nearest emergency room. In either case, bring along the substance's original container so the ingredients can be confirmed from the label.
- If the poison control center has been called, follow their immediate suggestions first, then bring the child and the container to the office for evaluation.
- If pills, nonpetroleum substances, or noncorrosives were ingested, the parent may induce vomiting with syrup of ipecac: For a child 1 to 4 years of age, administer 1 tablespoon (3 teaspoons) after giving 4 to 8 ounces (½ to 1 cup) of warm water. Repeat in 20 minutes if vomiting has not occurred. For an infant of 9 to 12 months, give 4 ounces (½ cup) of water followed by 2 teaspoons of syrup of ipecac. (See note in Telephone Decision Guidelines, question 4, about antiemetic pills and liquids.) Certain ingestions do not require a visit to the office.
- If corrosives (lye) or hydrocarbons (kerosene, furniture polish) were ingested, do not induce vomiting. Take the child and the container to the emergency room immediately. **In a true emergency, an ambulance should be summoned.**

Ingestions That May Be Managed Conservatively at Home

Sometimes there is no immediate need to bring the child to the office unless symptoms are present. The case should be reported to the clinician.

- **Coins** and smooth metallic objects, if there is no vomiting, abdominal pain, coughing, respiratory distress, or cyanosis. If the object contains lead or if any of these symptoms are occurring, the child should be seen at once and an x-ray obtained.
- **Small nonmetallic toys** and parts of toys, with the same exceptions as for coins.
- **Cosmetics,** such as powders or creams. If nail polish remover or hair dye, the child and the container should be brought in.
- **Bleaches** (e.g., Clorox) may cause oral and esophageal burns if in concentrated form. Cases should be judged on an individual basis.
- **Mercury** (metallic) from broken thermometers.
- **Vitamin pills** that **definitely** contain no iron.
- **Birth control pills** (fewer than 6 pills).

CHAPTER 24

■ ■ ■ ■ ■ ■ ■ ■ ■ ■ ■ ■ ■ ■
■
■
■
■
Rashes

Rashes usually should not be diagnosed over the telephone. One look is worth a thousand words. It is simply easier, quicker, and much more accurate to diagnose a rash after a proper examination. There are some important exceptions, however. Chickenpox, for example, is an illness most clinicians would prefer to keep out of the office because of the risk of contagion to other patients. Some skin conditions, such as eczema or diaper rash, may have been previously diagnosed and the parent is simply calling to request more medication. And occasionally a reliable parent can assume some of the responsibility for diagnosis, as when one child has been in to see the clinician with a plantar wart, and later another child in the family develops the same kind of lesion.

> The main role of telephone advice for rashes is clearly not diagnosis, but the dissemination of patient education information about:
> - Incubation period and duration of contagion
> - Possible complications, such as secondary infection
> - Treatment for relief of symptoms
> - Follow-up expectations and instructions

Skin disorders collectively are one of the most common reasons why parents call a clinician's office. For training purposes, this chapter will discuss in alphabetical order a number of rashes that together seem to generate most phone encounters: chickenpox, diaper rash, drug rashes, eczema, impetigo, petechiae, poison ivy, scarlatina, and warts. See Chapter 51 for a discussion of lice.

Chickenpox

There are more calls about chickenpox than for most other rashes. As already mentioned, it is best to try to avoid an office visit, but the child should be seen if:
- There is doubt about the diagnosis.
- The child appears very ill.
- The parent is anxious.
- There is a possible complication, such as ear or eye infection, pneumonia, brain involvement, or secondary bacterial infection of one of the skin lesions. The most serious of these secondary infections is the "flesh-eating strep," which is increased in cases of chickenpox.

> The characteristics of chickenpox include:
> - Multiple small blisters (vesicles) on a red base, often preceded by red, raised bumps (papules)

- Location of pox at the outset mainly on the chest, back, and stomach
- Lesions that occur in clusters so that some clusters contain fresh lesions while others are older, with black crusts already forming
- An incubation period of 11 to 21 days

Nonspecific symptoms of fever, listlessness, or decreased appetite can precede the rash by 1 to 2 days. The rash begins suddenly, with crops of raised red lesions that quickly form clear blisters on a red base. The contents of the blister become cloudy and then it ruptures, becoming scabbed or crusted over. Usually crops continue to erupt for 3 or 4 days. When the entire rash is scabbed over, the child is no longer contagious. The rash also may involve mucous membranes (mouth, genitals), where shallow ulcers form. The severity of the disease varies from a few lesions with little sign of illness to a widespread rash with high temperatures (102°F to 105°F). The duration ranges between 5 and 14 days, the average being about 7 days.

Treatment is directed at making the child comfortable by reducing itching, pain, and fever. The risk of secondary infection from scratching can be minimized by keeping the child's nails short and clean. Secondary bacterial infection is treated with oral antibiotics. Symptoms are managed by the liberal use of tub soaks with oatmeal or bath oils and using acetaminophen for fever and antihistamines for mild sedation and the relief of itching.

A chickenpox vaccine is now available and recommended as a routine immunization for children older than 12 months.

Diaper Rash

Diaper rash has several causes. Most rashes in the diaper area are caused by the wetness and irritation of moist diapers rubbing against the skin. Treatment consists of air-drying the skin (which can be speeded up by using a blow dryer), changing diapers frequently, and applying a protective barrier like Desitin, vitamin A and D ointment, or petroleum jelly (Vaseline). Diaper rash may become secondarily infected with bacteria or yeast. The most common secondary infection is with the yeast Candida, which also causes oral thrush and vaginitis. Whenever a diaper rash is reported to get worse or look infected, the child should be seen the same day.

Drug Rashes

When a child who is taking a medication develops a rash, it is important to rule out allergy to the drug, which is more likely to be the explanation if true hives are present. Between 5 and 10% of children taking amoxicillin develop a nonallergic rash, which is flat, pink, and not itchy. It usually lasts 3 to 4 days and requires no treatment.

In most instances, the child should be given an office appointment so the nature of the rash can be documented for future reference, or the call should be referred to the clinician for a final decision. The medication should be discontinued until the child is seen or the parent speaks to the clinician.

Eczema

Eczema, sometimes called atopic dermatitis, is a specific type of inflammation of the skin that occurs in children who have a genetic tendency toward allergy. The skin in eczema is red, swollen, itchy, and often weeping with crusts and scales. The creases of the elbow and behind the knee are frequently involved. Because of scratching, eczema frequently becomes secondarily infected.

There is a close association between eczema and other forms of allergy, like hay fever and asthma. Children with eczema have very sensitive skin, which reacts to stimuli such as dryness and certain types of fabric. In most children, the eczema either disappears or markedly improves by 5 years of age.

Any patient with a rash that seems to be eczema should be seen for treatment and have a full discussion with the clinician to promote a better understanding of this chronic disorder and its implications.

Impetigo

What Is It? Where Does It Come From?

Impetigo is a common skin infection that occurs in many children and adults. It usually starts when there is a break in the skin's surface from a mosquito bite, scratch, or irritation from a runny nose. Bacteria (most commonly Streptococcus or Staphylococcus species) are then introduced, often by scratching. When the child scratches or rubs the lesion, the bacteria get on the fingers, which then spread the infection to other areas or to someone else. Bacteria can be cultured from the lesions, but usually routine cultures are not indicated because of the expense and the ease of visual diagnosis.

How Is It Recognized?

Although impetigo is relatively common, many people are unfamiliar with its appearance. The lesions usually begin as small red bumps but soon enlarge, become moist-looking, and then develop yellowish crusts or scabs on a red base. When caused by Staphylococcus, the lesions generally appear as large, flat blisters filled with a milky fluid. These blisters can rupture, leaving raw areas. This form is often seen in infants but also can appear in older children and adults. Impetigo is most common during the summer.

The most common locations for impetigo are just below the nostrils and on the chin and extremities. Lesions vary in size from approximately ¼ inch to several inches in diameter.

Is It Contagious?

Impetigo is contagious. Contaminated washcloths and clothing should be washed with either Lysol or Clorox. Children should be kept out of school or day care until antibiotic treatment has been given for 24 to 36 hours.

Treatment

The most successful treatment for impetigo is an oral antibiotic. Even small lesions require treatment. If there are only one or two very small lesions, topical treatment can be tried, including washing with antibacterial soap and applying Bacitracin or Neosporin ointment, which can be obtained without a prescription. Patients may start topical therapy (three to four times a day for a week) when there is a question of an early infection, but if new lesions appear or the initial lesion enlarges, the child should be seen in the office and considered for oral antibiotic therapy.

Potential Complications

The treatment may appear overly aggressive for a relatively mild skin disorder, but there are two important reasons to treat impetigo promptly. First, it does not respond well to local treatment and may spread to involve large areas of skin and underlying tissues. Second, skin infections caused by certain strains of streptococcus bacteria occasionally can lead to glomerulonephritis, a kidney disorder characterized by bloody urine. (The same group A, beta-hemolytic strep that causes sore throats is the organism that causes impetigo.) It is hoped that the kidney disease will be prevented by prompt therapy.

Petechiae

Petechiae are lesions caused by bleeding into the skin. Unlike a bruise, a petechia is a tiny, pinpoint red dot. Unlike most red rashes, a petechia will not blanch. (Place one thumb on each side of the lesion, press, and spread apart. A petechia will stay red; the redness of most other red rashes will disappear.) Petechiae may appear suddenly in crops or clusters on any part of the body.

Any child with petechiae should be seen immediately because they sometimes signify a serious bloodstream infection. There are a number of less serious causes for petechiae, but an evaluation in the office is needed for specific diagnosis.

Poison Ivy

Poison ivy is a form of contact dermatitis, which means that a substance has touched the skin and produced a very itchy rash—usually red, with tiny blisters. The rashes of poison ivy, oak, and sumac are indistinguishable. These plants are easily recognized and bloom in profusion during the summer and fall. Children should be taught to identify poison ivy, by far the most common problem.

If a child has been in contact with poison ivy, immediate thorough cleansing with soap and water can lessen the dermatitis. Lotions such as calamine dry the lesions and help relieve discomfort. Benadryl, an antihistamine, can also be used if the itching is troublesome. Rarely, cortisone medication (prednisone) is needed to treat the rash and swelling. If the rash covers a large portion of the body, if it seems to be infected, if the eyes are swollen, or if the discomfort is extreme, the child should be seen.

Scarlatina

Scarlatina, or scarlet fever, is a strep throat plus a rash that is actually caused by an allergic reaction to the "strep" germ. It does not have the serious implications that it had in the era before antibiotics and is really no different from strep tonsillitis, aside from the rash. The rash is very characteristic: tiny, raised bumps that are very red and feel rough like sandpaper when they are gently rubbed. The skin looks like a sunburn with goose bumps and often peels in about 7 to 10 days. Children with this kind of rash need a same-day appointment. Treatment with antibiotics is highly effective.

Warts

Warts are caused by a viral infection of the skin. Unfortunately, warts are often misunderstood and cause considerable emotional distress. Warts are not a threat to a patient's health. They often disappear without treatment, but this may take several years. In the meantime, the patient may acquire additional warts by self-inoculation of the virus from existing warts or may spread the virus to other susceptible individuals.

Treatment of warts should be appropriate to the age of the child and the size and location of the wart. Because of the discomfort of treatment and the difficulty of getting full cooperation, children under 6 should not be treated unless there are special circumstances such as pain, bleeding, or a location on the face or close to the fingernail. Plantar warts, located on the bottom of the foot, should be removed because they are almost always quite painful. Children who are very young, who have warts that are complicated or widespread or who have a potential for a poor cosmetic result should be referred to a dermatologist, but these referrals should be rare. If parents are reassured that warts are benign and that the long-term cosmetic results are best if the wart is allowed to go away spontaneously, they usually are willing to take a conservative approach.

When home methods of treatment are prescribed, such as 40% salicylic acid plaster or Duofilm (salicylic acid 17% and lactic acid 17% in flexible collodion), one should be specific about the method of application. Caution should be used to avoid applying these substances to the adjacent normal skin. Always discuss the size of the area to be treated, frequency of application, duration of treatment, and possible complications, such as irritant dermatitis and infection. The possibility of bacterial infection should not be overlooked. Any break in the skin serves as a source of entry for bacteria. Good skin hygiene should be emphasized and topical antibiotics used when appropriate.

TELEPHONE DECISION GUIDELINES

RASHES

Question	To See Clinician If . . .	When
1. Patient's name, telephone number, age	All children with unexplained rashes should be seen the same or next day.	8
2. Please describe the rash. Location? How long has it been present?	Blister on a red base, or clusters of blisters, some of which may be crusted.	See question 4
	Looks like an irritation in the diaper area.	See question 7
	Looks crusted, oozing, and infected (suggests impetigo, especially if located around the nostrils).	8
	Itches, weeps clear liquid, or appears in lines (suggests poison ivy).	8
	Looks like sunburn, feels slightly rough like sandpaper; located mainly in skin creases such as arm, groin, neck, armpit (suggests scarlatina).	8
3. Any associated symptoms? Fever? Sore throat? Earache?	Yes, any of these.	8

Chickenpox

Question	To See Clinician If . . .	When
4. Is the parent sure it's chickenpox (previous experience, recent exposure)?	Yes—home management advice is appropriate (but see questions 5 and 6). No (see questions 5 and 6).	8
5. Does the child appear very ill?	Yes.	2
6. Does the blister appear very red and rapidly enlarging, with increasing pain?	Yes (rule out serious secondary infection).	2

Diaper Rash

Question	To See Clinician If . . .	When
7. Is the rash spreading, getting worse, and not responding to diaper rash medication?	Begin with home management advice, but if rash worsens, child should be seen to rule out a fungal infection.	8

EMS = Activate EMS System		24-72 = Appointment within 3 days	
2 = See ASAP (within 1–2 hours)		72+ = Appointment in 4 days or more	
8 = See same day			

High priority items appear in color.

P
E
D
I
A
T
R
I
C

ADVICE

Under certain circumstances, as discussed earlier in the chapter, home management advice for specific rashes may be appropriate. Following is advice for these conditions:

Chickenpox

- Use acetaminophen (Tylenol) as needed for fever and discomfort. Do not give aspirin.
- Follow advice under Poison Ivy to manage itching and scratching.

Uncomplicated Diaper Rash

- Bathe with warm water.
- Dry thoroughly with a towel or a blow-dryer held 8 to 10 inches from the body and set on low heat to avoid burns.
- Leave the diaper area exposed to air for prolonged periods (½ to 1 hour) during the day, such as during naps. Air is the best remedy.
- Change diapers frequently.
- Apply a thick coat of petroleum jelly (Vaseline), vitamin A and D ointment, or Desitin after each cleansing.

Poison Ivy

- Apply calamine lotion with a cotton ball.
- Give the child a tub bath with either Alpha Keri bath oil or Aveeno oatmeal bath (2 cups added to lukewarm bath water).
- For itching, give an antihistamine, Chlor-Trimeton or Benadryl, as shown in Table 24–1. Reduce the dose if the child becomes too drowsy. No prescription is needed.
- Cut the child's fingernails as short as possible and clean them with a nailbrush.

Plantar Warts

These painful warts can be treated with a 40% salicylic acid plaster (medicine incorporated into a sheet of tape):

- Apply the plaster after a bath or shower.
- Cut the plaster to the exact outline of the wart. Do not apply it to normal skin.
- The plaster will not remain attached unless it is covered with adhesive tape. Use a strip long enough to attach the plaster firmly.
- Leave the plaster in place for 24 hours. Remove it before the child takes a bath or shower and apply a fresh plaster afterward.
- If the skin becomes irritated or uncomfortable, leave the plaster off for 2 or 3 days.
- Do not use a plaster if the wart appears infected. Call for an appointment.
- Remember that the wart might persist for months. Be patient.

TABLE 24-1	Antihistamine Treatment for Itch and Allergy	
Age	**Chlor-Trimeton Syrup (2 mg/tsp) or Tablet (4 mg/tab)**	**Benadryl Elixir (12.5 mg/tsp) or Tablet (25 mg/tab)**
Under 1 year	Not recommended unless specified by clinician	Not recommended unless specified by clinician
1–5 years	½ tsp three or four times daily	½–1 tsp three or four times daily
6–12 years	1 tsp three or four times daily	1–1½ tsp three or four times daily
Over 12 years	2 tsp or 1 tablet three times daily	2 tsp or 1 tablet every 4–6 hours (maximum 3–4 tablets/day)

CHAPTER 25

. . . .
:
:
:   Sore Throat
:

Infection of the tonsils and throat (pharynx) is the major cause of a sore throat. The medical terms that describe the infection include tonsillitis, pharyngitis, and pharyngo-tonsillitis. Most infections involve both the tonsils and the pharynx, which can be viewed as a combined anatomical unit.

Infections of the throat may be caused by both viruses and bacteria.

> The common bacterial cause of sore throats is the "strep" germ, an abbreviated term for the bacteria called group A beta-hemolytic Streptococcus (GABHS). For practical purposes, the major question to answer about a throat infection is "Is it strep or not?"

Most infections are viral; symptoms subside spontaneously and antibiotics are not effective. Unfortunately, clinical inspection of the throat alone cannot determine whether the infection is viral or bacterial, so a throat culture or a rapid strep test, performed and interpreted by trained personnel, is the mainstay of deciding between viral and strep infections.

Bacterial causes other than strep do not have to be considered unless there are special reasons. The primary purpose of identifying GABHS is to avoid complications such as rheumatic fever (arthritis and heart problems) and nephritis (bleeding into the kidney and urine, associated with kidney failure), which can occur as a delayed reaction if the infection is not treated properly. Treatment of strep throat consists of antibiotics, usually penicillin if there is no allergy to this drug.

The response to treatment for strep is usually rapid and successful. Occasionally the strep survives treatment and symptoms recur. Parents should not become overly frustrated if this occurs. The cause for the recurrence can usually be determined and the problem resolved. Discussion between parent and clinician may focus on subjects such as why some children may not absorb oral antibiotics well enough from the stomach, and therefore require injections rather than oral medication; whether the child is actually taking all of the medicine (compliance); spreading of the strep germ within a family (ping-pong effect); when it may be appropriate for other family members to be cultured (rarely); the carrier state (strep in the throat but no symptoms or signs); and lastly, the role of tonsillectomy in the management of recurrent streptococcal throat infections. Close communication between the parent and the clinician is needed to avoid misinterpretation about the reason for recurrent throat infections and their significance. Fortunately, very few children present this problem. The role of the telephone triage staff person is to recognize the nature of the problem for those who do and refer them to the clinician.

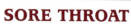

TELEPHONE DECISION GUIDELINES

SORE THROAT

Question	To See Clinician If . . .	When
1. Patient's name, telephone number, age	Age under 4 years	8
2. Is the child drooling or having difficulty breathing?	Yes	2
3. Is the child acting particularly ill?	Yes	2
4. Does the child have a stiff neck?	Yes	2
5. Does the child have a rash, headache, or stomachache?	Yes	2
6. Is the pain severe?	Yes	2
7. Does the child have any serious or chronic illness?	Yes—diabetes, asthma, kidney disease, congenital heart disease, etc.	2
8. If the child has a rash, does it look like sunburn?	Yes (rule out scarlatina)	8
9. Has the child had many sore throats or strep infections before?	Yes	8
10. How long has the child had the sore throat? Is it only sore in the morning or all the time?	More than 12 hours and continuous	8
11. Does the child have a fever?	Yes, above 101°F	8
12. Are the glands in the neck swollen or tender?	Yes	8

EMS	= Activate EMS SYSTEM	24-72	= Appointment within 3 days
2	= See ASAP (within 1–2 hours)	72+	= Appointment in 4 days or more
8	= See same day		

High priority items appear in color.

ADVICE

If the child has awakened with a sore throat in the morning and is otherwise well, without fever, or possibly has a mild cold associated with a sore throat, advise the parent to give the child more fluids to drink and humidify the room (particularly if the child is a mouth breather). If the sore throat goes away after a few hours, no further treatment will be necessary. The parent should call back if the sore throat worsens or persists.

To relieve symptoms, recommend the following:

- Encourage fluids such as water, apple juice, popsicles, soup, or Jell-O. Avoid acids like orange juice.
- Use acetaminophen (Tylenol) or children's ibuprofen for relief of pain or fever. See Tables 18–1 and 18–2 (pp. 79–80) for dosages.
- A mixture of tea, lemon, and honey may be soothing.
- Children who are old enough can gargle with weak, warm salt water (add ¼ teaspoon to 4 ounces of warm water) for additional relief if needed.
- Older children also can suck on hard candy. It is a choking hazard for toddlers.

CHAPTER 26

■ ■ ■ ■ ■ ■ ■ ■ ■ ■ ■ ■ ■ ■

Strains and Sprains

Minor orthopedic trauma prompts a large number of phone calls to the pediatrician or family practitioner. Most of these injuries involve muscle strains or ligamentous sprains, usually involving the knee or ankle, or fractures. Whenever a large number of adolescents are involved in sports, the incidence of these injuries will be even greater.

Muscle strains are usually quite painful but not serious. The role of telephone triage is to rule out the possibility that the strain is actually something more serious, like a fracture or joint problem. Most of these strained muscles can be traced to the child's starting a new sport and "pulling" a muscle while running or overexerting in gym class, when the soreness is more likely to appear the next day. If there is any doubt, the child should be examined, but if the explanation for the muscle strain is clear-cut, advice can be given on the telephone for home management (heat, acetaminophen or ibuprofen, and rest), which should remedy the situation in a short time.

Sprains are more serious and represent damage to the ligaments that attach to the bones of a joint. They are produced by accidents that force the joint into an abnormal position. Ligaments surrounding any joint can be stretched in a mild sprain and torn or even separated from the bone in a more severe injury. The amount of pain and the degree of swelling can be comparable to what is seen with a fracture. Badly sprained ankles are the most common example.

Treatment of a sprain will depend on the extent of injury. For mild sprains, ice, compression, and elevation (ICE) are helpful, and the sprain usually is resolved within a few days. More severe sprains may require casting, crutches, or even surgery in extreme cases.

> All but the most minor sprains should be examined, because failure to treat the sprain properly at the onset could result in a longer period of discomfort and a less satisfactory long-term outcome.

STRAINS AND SPRAINS

Question	To See Clinician If . . .	When
1. Patient's name, telephone number, age		
2. What part of the body was injured? Is there much pain?	**Any joint, if at all painful** **A muscle, only if pain is severe**	2
3. Is the area red, warm, or swollen?	**Yes**	2
4. Does the child have a fever or appear ill?	Yes to either	8

EMS = Activate EMS SYSTEM		24-72 = Appointment within 3 days	
2 = See ASAP (within 1–2 hours)		72+ = Appointment in 4 days or more	
8 = See same day			

High priority items appear in color.

ADVICE

If the history clearly indicates a pulled or strained muscle only and there are no complicating factors, home management can be carried out as follows:

- Rest.
- Heat (heating pad or hot water bag) for 15 minutes four times a day until improved.
- Acetaminophen (Tylenol) or ibuprofen (Advil, Motrin) for pain.
- Call back if the symptoms worsen or do not improve or if the pain persists after 3 days of treatment.

In general, all painful joints should be examined. Home management can be tried, however, for a minimal twist of the ankle that is only slightly uncomfortable, as long as there is no swelling and the parent is not anxious:

- Wrap an ice-filled plastic bag in a towel and place it on the ankle for 20 minutes of each hour for the first 4 hours after the injury.
- Compress the ankle by wrapping an Ace bandage around it. Begin at the bottom of the foot, making the first wind toward the outside of the foot and moving upward. Do not stretch the bandage or make it too tight. The foot should feel comfortable after it is wrapped. The bandage can be kept on as long as it helps.
- Elevate the foot whenever possible as long as there is pain.
- Give acetaminophen (Tylenol) or ibuprofen (Advil, Motrin) for pain.
- Increase the use of the foot gradually. Call back if it does not improve within 2 or 3 days.

CHAPTER 27

▪ ▪ ▪ ▪ ▪ ▪ ▪ ▪ ▪ ▪ ▪ ▪ ▪ ▪

Urinary Burning and Frequency

The complaint of burning on urination (dysuria) and frequency of urination is much more common in girls and should always raise the concern of a urinary tract infection (UTI). Another cause in girls is a vaginal infection (with or without a discharge), which irritates the urinary outlet. Bubble baths also may irritate the urethra and should be discouraged. Also, with pinworm infection, the worms may crawl from the anus to the vagina and irritate the vagina, causing burning. Treatment for both the pinworms and the vaginal inflammation is indicated.

Urinary Tract Infection

UTI is a more serious cause of dysuria and frequency. It is one of the most common and important forms of bacterial infection in childhood. The urinary tract includes the kidneys, ureters, bladder, and urethra. In children older than 1 year, UTI affects 10 times more girls than boys. In addition to urinary burning and frequency, symptoms can include the recent onset of bedwetting, abdominal pain, chronic diarrhea, chills, and fever.

> Some urinary tract infections cause few or no symptoms. The urine culture is the critical diagnostic test. The culture determines whether infection is present, what bacteria are causing the infection, and the best drugs to use to treat it.

Collecting Urine for the Urine Culture

Parents must be carefully instructed in the method for obtaining a "clean-catch" urine specimen at home. A contaminated culture (which will need to be repeated) can be avoided by proper cleansing, proper collection, and prompt delivery of the urine specimen to the laboratory. Thorough cleansing of the urethral opening is essential. The middle of the urine stream, if possible, should be obtained in a sterile container. The urine should be refrigerated immediately and delivered to the office or laboratory not more than 2 hours after collection. The longer the delay, the more chance for contamination. Urinary catheterization, or a suprapubic bladder tap in young infants, may be recommended.

Causes of Urinary Tract Infection

Approximately one-third of girls and the majority of boys who have a urinary tract infection will have a demonstrable cause for the infection:

- **Obstruction:** a narrowing of the urinary tract in any of its locations
- **Reflux:** a back-up of urine from the bladder into the ureters

- **Anomalies:** congenital abnormalities of the kidneys or urinary tract (for example, a horseshoe-shaped kidney)

All of these can lead to pyelonephritis, scarring of the kidney, as a result of long-standing or recurrent infections. Many children whose urinary tracts appear normal by x-ray nevertheless have recurrent UTI. The cause in these children remains unknown.

Pain on Urination in the Male

Urinary tract infection is much less common in boys. If a negative urinalysis and urine culture rules out UTI in a boy who complains of burning on urination, other causes for the pain should be sought. One is local irritation at the tip of the penis, sometimes associated with masturbation. In adolescents, infection of the urethra by a variety of bacteria is a major cause. Sexually transmitted diseases (STDs) should be ruled out by appropriate tests. STDs are not always accompanied by a discharge from the penis. All boys with dysuria should be given a same-day appointment.

Frequency without Dysuria

Unusually frequent (but painless) passing of large volumes of urine (polyuria) should suggest the possibility of diabetes.

Other cardinal symptoms of diabetes include intense thirst (polydipsia), increased appetite, and weight loss. There also may be recent onset of bedwetting. All patients with these symptoms should be seen as soon as possible for a physical examination and urinalysis.

URINARY BURNING AND FREQUENCY

Question	To See Clinician If . . .	When
1. Patient's name, telephone number, age		
2. Does the child appear ill?	**Yes.**	2
3. Does the child have a fever?	**Yes.**	2
4. How long has the child had pain on urination?	More than 24 hours.	8
5. Has the child had a urinary tract infection in the past?	Yes.	8
6. Does the child have urinary frequency without pain?	Yes.	8
7. (If a girl) Is there a vaginal discharge?	Yes.	8
8. (If a girl) Does the child have itching around her rectum?	Yes.	8
9. Is there redness or irritation • (If a boy) at the tip of the penis? • (If a girl) near the vagina?	Home advice appropriate initially. Child should be seen if symptoms persist after ointment is used.	8
10. Does the child bathe with bubble bath?	Advise discontinuing bubble bath. Parent should bring urine specimen.	

EMS	= Activate EMS SYSTEM	24-72	= Appointment within 3 days
2	= See ASAP (within 1–2 hours)	72+	= Appointment in 4 days or more
8	= See same day		

High priority items appear in color.

ADVICE

If the child appears well and has no fever, and mild symptoms have been present for less than 24 hours:

- Bring a urine specimen to the office for urinalysis and urine culture. (See instructions below.)
- Place child in sitz bath of plain warm water for relief of pain and relaxation.
- The child may void directly into water.
- If redness is visible at the tip of a boy's penis, put petroleum jelly (Vaseline) or A and D Ointment on the area of irritation. Call office for appointment if symptoms persist or worsen.
- Call the office in 24 hours for urine culture results and to report the effect of treatment on the symptoms. If the child is worse or the urine test is abnormal, schedule an appointment for the same day.

Collecting a Proper Urine Specimen at Home

1. Boil a small jar and its lid for 20 minutes and air-cool it.
2. Completely remove the child's pants and panties and have the child sit straddling the toilet.
3. Wash the genitalia gently with soap and water.
4. Using the sterile jar, try to catch the middle of the urine stream if at all possible.
5. Always refrigerate the specimen immediately. Bring it to the office or lab as quickly as possible, preferably within 2 hours.

CHAPTER 28

■ ■ ■ ■ ■ ■ ■ ■ ■ ■ ■ ■ ■ ■

Vomiting

Vomiting can occur with diarrhea or alone. One of the most common causes of vomiting is a viral infection ("stomach flu"), but there are many other causes, which may vary with the age of the child. In infancy the reasons for vomiting range from simple overfeeding and milk protein intolerance to more serious reasons such as pyloric stenosis, intestinal obstruction, gastroesophageal reflux, and sepsis. The smaller the infant, the greater the likelihood of dehydration. In older children the causes for vomiting include gastroenteritis, hepatitis, migraine, and reactions to drugs or toxic agents. In adolescence, vomiting may be associated with pregnancy, anorexia, or bulimia.

If vomiting, with or without fever, has persisted for over 24 hours, an examination is indicated. One of the functions of telephone triage for children who are vomiting is to attempt to evaluate whether the child is dehydrated based on whether the child is lethargic, when the child last urinated, and whether the inside of the cheeks and lips is moist or dry. If the patient can tolerate small sips of fluid or ice chips, oral rehydration should be attempted.

> The signs of dehydration include:
> - Listlessness
> - Dry tongue and inner cheek
> - Tears absent when crying
> - Sunken eyeballs
> - No urination in the past 8 to 10 hours

If a small child or infant refuses sips of fluid and feedings, a visit is indicated. A visit is also indicated when colicky abdominal pain is associated with the vomiting.

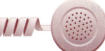

TELEPHONE DECISION GUIDELINES

VOMITING

Question	To See Clinician If . . .	When
1. Patient's name, telephone number, age	Per clinician preference	
2. Does the child appear unusually ill?	Yes	2
3. Does the child seem dehydrated? Is the mouth moist? When did the child last urinate?	Dehydration suspected—dry mouth, no urination for 8 to 10 hours, listless, etc.	2
4. Does the child have other symptoms besides vomiting?		
• Severe headache or stiff neck?	Yes	2
• Abdominal pain?	Yes	2
• Pain or burning on urination?	Yes	2
• Excessive irritability, listlessness, or mental confusion?	Yes	2
• Earache, cold, or sore throat?	Yes	2
• Severe diarrhea?	Yes (see Chapter 15, Diarrhea)	2
• Any blood in the vomitus?	Yes	2
• Breathing hard or fast?	Yes	2
• Any exposure to a poisonous substance?	Yes	2
• Fever?	Yes, for more than 24 hours	8
5. How long has the child been vomiting? What has the child eaten during that time?	More than 24 hours without improvement while on a clear liquid diet	8
6. How many times has the child vomited?	More than three times in past 6 hours; not taking fluid by mouth	8
7. Does the child have any serious or chronic illness?	Yes—diabetes, asthma, etc.	8
8. Is the child receiving any medication?	Yes, a drug that may cause vomiting (e.g., erythromycin) or a drug that is needed daily (e.g., amoxicillin for earache)	8

EMS	= Activate EMS SYSTEM	24-72	= Appointment within 3 days
2	= See ASAP (within 1–2 hours)	72+	= Appointment in 4 days or more
8	= See same day		

High priority items appear in color.

TELEPHONE DECISION GUIDELINES /////////////

WOUNDS

Question	To See Clinician If . . .	When
1. Patient's name, telephone number, age	Age under 1 year.	2
2. Is the wound still bleeding? Have you applied pressure to it?	Wound still bleeding after 10 minutes of direct, firm pressure with a clean cloth.	EMS

Puncture Wound

Question	To See Clinician If . . .	When
3. When and how did the wound occur? (e.g., Was it rusty nail? Was it inside or outside the house?)	Wound may be contaminated.	2
4. Is the wound very deep?	Yes.	2
5. Is foreign material visible in the wound?	Yes.	2
6. Are there any signs of infection in the area, such as redness, swelling, red streaks extending from the wound, discharge or pus draining from the wound?	Yes, any of these.	8
7. Has the child had the complete primary series of tetanus shots? (three or more)	No.	8
8. When was the last tetanus booster?	More than 10 years ago.	8
9. Have you cleaned the wound thoroughly?	No—Give advice for home treatment.	

Laceration (Cut)

Question	To See Clinician If . . .	When
10. Does the cut look bad? Is it gaping or split open? Is it jagged or deep?	Yes—anything more than a small scratch.	2
11. Go back to questions 6–9.		

EMS = Activate EMS SYSTEM   24-72 = Appointment within 3 days

2 = See ASAP (within 1–2 hours)   72+ = Appointment in 4 days or more

8 = See same day

High priority items appear in color.

ADVICE

Apply direct pressure firmly for 10 minutes to stop any bleeding. Lacerations should be flushed with tap water, and then firm pressure should be applied with a clean cloth to control bleeding before starting out for the office or emergency room.

Puncture wounds and abrasions should be washed very thoroughly, as follows:

1. Flush with cool water running from the tap.
2. Scrub gently with soap and water, using a soft washcloth, and rinse.
3. Apply an antiseptic such as 3% hydrogen peroxide, or mercurochrome.
4. Dry and cover with a Band-Aid or sterile gauze if the wound is in an area that is likely to get dirty. Use a nonstick dressing for a large abrasion.
5. Observe daily for any signs of local infection or signs of illness.

TELEPHONE TRIAGE: SYMPTOMS IN ADULTS

CHAPTER 30

Abdominal Pain

Jeannette M. Shorey, MD

Abdominal pain is a symptom. It has many possible sources, with consequences for the patient ranging from transient discomfort to life-threatening illness. The pain, as well as other accompanying signs and symptoms, may be dramatic or subtle, and similar patterns can be produced by different diseases. Diagnosing the cause of abdominal pain thus is one of the most challenging tasks a clinician must perform.

> When a patient calls with abdominal pain, the threshold for recommending a visit with a clinician for a thorough history and physical examination should be low. The challenge to the telephone triage staff is largely a matter of determining when that visit can safely take place.

Abdominal pain that has begun in recent hours usually deserves evaluation more promptly than pain that has been around for several days, weeks, or months. The severity of the patient's pain and other significant medical problems will help determine how quickly the patient should be seen.

Appropriate management of abdominal pain requires a specific diagnosis. Sometimes a patient can describe symptoms clearly enough that experienced telephone staff can feel confident about the diagnosis. For example, if a mother with a son in nursery school who had similar symptoms yesterday reports that she now has low-grade fever, nausea, and intermittent crampy abdominal pain followed by vomiting of bile or the passage of watery, brown diarrhea, the diagnosis of gastroenteritis is almost certain. If this mother can drink and keep down fluids, she can safely be advised to gently "push fluids," take aspirin or acetaminophen (Tylenol) to control her fever and rest as much as possible—with other family members taking care of the child, if possible. All family members should be told to practice careful hand washing, and the patient should call back if symptoms worsen or do not resolve within 48 hours. Contrast that story with a case of severe abdominal pain in an elderly person who has other significant medical problems and a symptom complex that is less clear. No one should attempt to manage this patient by phone. The patient must be advised to obtain care promptly from a clinician and should be helped with an appointment or transportation assistance if needed.

Abdominal pain can be caused by a wide range of both common and rare disorders. Some, such as intestinal infections, peptic ulcer, appendicitis, or ectopic pregnancy, are centered in the abdomen itself. Pain in the abdomen also may be referred from other sources such as pneumonia in the chest, may have a metabolic cause such as lead poisoning, may be caused by injury to the nervous system, or may have a psychological basis.

The following key signs and symptoms should compel telephone triage staff to advise an evaluation by a clinician:

- Severe, unremitting, constant pain or severe waves of colicky pain
- Symptoms such as faintness, weakness, clamminess, or sweating, which may indicate shock
- Chest pain or shortness of breath
- Bloody or tarry stool
- Trauma
- Fever greater than 101°F
- A missed menstrual period or two
- Pregnancy
- Unremittting vomiting or severe constipation
- Serious medical illness such as diabetes mellitus, coronary artery disease, chronic obstructive pulmonary disease, chronic renal failure, or immunosuppressive illnesses like malignancies, HIV infection, and AIDS
- Chronic use of oral steroid medications (**not** modest doses of inhaled steroids for asthma or rhinitis)
- Back pain
- Urinary symptoms such as urgency, frequency, or blood in the urine
- Cough, fever, and sputum production

This list is lengthy. It underscores the low threshold for advising patients with abdominal pain to seek evaluation by a clinician.

As illustrated earlier, however, in some cases home management can be advised. Patients who are generally healthy at baseline and describe mild symptoms of abdominal pain without any of the other problems just listed can be advised to rest, maintain good fluid intake, try topical treatments like a heating pad or warm bath, and call back if the symptoms worsen or fail to resolve.

ABDOMINAL PAIN

Question	To See Clinician If . . .	When
1. Patient's name, age, telephone number		
2. Is the pain severe and persistent? Did it begin suddenly?	Yes. (Consult clinician about urgency of visit if time permits.)	EMS
3. Do you feel dizzy, clammy, sweaty, or too weak to stand? (Or is the caller reporting a patient who has fainted?)	Yes.	EMS
4. Do you have shortness of breath or chest pain?	Yes.	EMS
5. (If the patient is female) Are you pregnant?	Yes.	EMS
6. Have you experienced a recent abdominal injury?	Yes.	EMS
7. Do you have bloody stools; black, tarry stools; or bleeding from the rectum?	Yes.	2
8. Do you have a fever higher than 101°F?	Yes.	2
9. Have you had kidney stones, gallstones, or sickle cell crisis that has caused similar pain in the past?	Yes.	2
10. (If the patient is female) Is the pain intense and associated with a missed menstrual period?	Yes.	2
11. (If the patient is male) Are your testicles painful?	Yes.	2
12. Are you diabetic?	Yes.	2
13. Do you take oral steroid medications?	Yes.	2
14. If the pain is severe, do you have frequent vomiting or severe constipation?	Yes.	2
15. If you are older than 50, is there back pain or history of severe atherosclerosis, heart attack, or stroke?	Yes.	2
16. Do you have urinary urgency, frequency, or blood in the urine?	Yes.	8
17. Do you have cough, fever, and sputum production?	Yes.	8

A
D
U
L
T

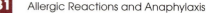

The symptoms of anaphylaxis may improve and later recur in about 20% of individuals, particularly those experiencing a severe episode. The late recurrence of symptoms in this biphasic pattern represents a late-phase reaction, not just inadequate therapy.

The most common cause of anaphylaxis is food allergy (especially involving peanuts, nuts, or seafood). Such allergies occur in about 30% of patients in most studies. Other common causes include Hymenoptera (bee, yellow jacket, and wasp) stings and fire-ant bites and drug allergy (especially involving antibiotics or nonsteroidal anti-inflammatory agents [NSAIDs]). In some populations, such as medical personnel or those who have had multiple surgeries, latex is a potential allergen. Less commonly, exercise may provoke anaphylaxis. In women, anaphylaxis may be particularly severe just before the menstrual period. No cause can be identified in a significant percentage of individuals.

Anaphylaxis may be confused with other conditions that share similar symptoms. These include panic attacks, vocal-cord dysfunction, acute urticaria or angioedema, vasodepressor reactions, mastocytosis, carcinoid syndrome, and C1 esterase inhibitor deficiency, a condition that may cause episodes of angioedema (swelling).

ALLERGIC REACTIONS AND ANAPHYLAXIS

Question	To See Clinician If . . .	When
1. Patient's name, age, telephone number	Anaphylaxis is always potentially life threatening. Emergency therapy is always indicated, even if symptoms are minor.	EMS
2. Have you experienced anaphylaxis before? If so, how severe was the episode?	Previous severe episodes, particularly those with airway obstruction and low blood pressure, suggest the potential for more severe recurrence.	EMS
3. Do you feel faint? (Or is the caller reporting a patient who is unconscious?)	Feeling faint or losing consciousness is particularly ominous. A patient who is unconscious should be placed flat on his or her back on a surface that is tilted with the head downward. If an epinephrine auto-injector (e.g., EpiPen) has previously been prescribed, it should be administered. Antihistamines are not the primary treatment of choice but may be helpful second-line drugs.	EMS
4. Are you alone?	Yes.	EMS
5. What other symptoms do you have? Hives? Swelling? Noisy or difficult breathing? Nausea? Vomiting? Diarrhea? How rapidly are they progressing?	A high-pitched, harsh sound during breathing (stridor) could represent airway obstruction that may progress to acute obstruction. See question 3 for treatment advice.	EMS
6. Are you taking a beta blocker, ACE inhibitor, MAO inhibitor, or tricyclic antidepressant?	If the patient is taking a tricyclic antidepressant (Tofranil, Elavil, Pamelor, etc.) or MAO inhibitor (Nardil, Parnate), the dose of epinephrine should be decreased.	EMS
7. What is the suspected cause of this event? Food (which)? Insect sting? Medication? Latex? Exercise? How long ago did the exposure or ingestion occur?	Note specifics and prior experience.	
8. Do you have any complicating medical disorder, such as cardiovascular or CNS disease?	Note specifics.	

EMS = Activate EMS SYSTEM	24-72 = Appointment within 3 days
2 = See ASAP (within 1–2 hours)	72+ = Appointment in 4 days or more
8 = See same day	

High priority items appear in color.

A
D
U
L
T

ADVICE

Do not try to manage any event at home regardless of how mild the episode appears. Even if the patient's past episodes were mild, subsequent attacks may be more severe. If a prior episode was severe, the likelihood of a similar recurrence is high. Therefore, emergent therapy is always indicated. It is particularly important to activate EMS as quickly as possible if

- The patient is alone.
- Symptoms suggest faintness or loss of consciousness.
- There are signs of airway obstruction, including stridor, hoarseness, wheezing, or difficulty in breathing.
- The patient has been taking a beta-blocking agent or ACE inhibitor.

If epinephrine is available, it should be administered. The sooner epinephrine is administered, the more likely the outcome will be satisfactory. Antihistamines are not the treatment of choice but may be of some benefit.

If the patient is wheezing, the use of a beta agonist inhaled bronchodilator (e.g., albuterol) may help to relieve airway obstruction. The patient should take two to four inhalations.

Because anaphylaxis may have two phases, initial relief of symptoms should not delay activation of EMS or emergent therapy. Patients or their companions should tell the emergency staff if the patient is taking a beta blocker, ACE inhibitor, MAO inhibitor, or tricyclic antidepressant. They also should try to identify the suspected cause of the anaphylaxis. If uncertain, they should try to outline in detail exposures, including food, medications, sting or bite, exercise activity, time during the menstrual cycle (for women), and any prior experience regarding anaphylaxis.

A
D
U
L
T

CHAPTER 32

■ ■ ■ ■ ■ ■ ■ ■ ■ ■ ■ ■ ■ ■
■
■
■
■
:

Back Pain

Robert H. Fletcher, MD, MSc

Nearly everyone experiences an acute attack of low back pain sometime in life. Most attacks are self-limited. Patients may need to see a physician, but special tests (such as x-rays) and referrals to specialists are rarely useful. The challenge in office practice is to reassure and relieve the symptoms of most patients, who will do well with this kind of care, while recognizing the few who need immediate, high-level attention.

Causes and Course

Low Back Strain

Most attacks of low back pain are caused by muscle spasm and strain of ligaments and other structures in and around the spine. The patient experiences the sudden onset of pain, often while lifting or moving awkwardly, and then finds it difficult to straighten up and move about freely. Sometimes the attacks come on overnight, for no apparent reason. Pain and tenderness are located in the low back, often on one side, and may spread to the hips and upper legs. Pain can be severe, even if the underlying cause is not serious.

This sort of garden-variety back pain usually improves quickly. Most attacks are gone in a few weeks no matter how they are treated. Studies have shown that the duration of symptoms is similar whether the care is from a primary care physician, orthopedic surgeon, or chiropractor. Visiting a chiropractor is safe and may make patients feel well looked-after, but chiropractic care will not shorten the episode. Referral to a specialist such as an orthopedic surgeon or neurosurgeon is useful only in severe cases, when there are specific signs and symptoms that suggest severe disease requiring surgery, as discussed later.

The usual treatment is over-the-counter pain medicines such as aspirin or ibuprofen (both to relieve pain itself and because pain causes spasm), hot or cold applications (there are two schools of thought), no heavy lifting, and usually time off work. Some clinicians prescribe muscle-relaxing drugs.

> Patients with low back strain are advised to find whatever position is comfortable for them; usually bed rest is no more helpful than limited activity.

Ruptured Disk

Sometimes low back pain is caused by rupture of one of the rubbery disks between the vertebrae; the disk pinches a nerve that is leaving the spinal canal on its way to the legs. The resulting pain, called **sciatica**, begins in the back but travels along the course of the nerve, typically down the back of the leg to the foot. This pain is made worse by bending over, leaning forward, and coughing. Weakness or numbness of the leg can also occur.

Even this kind of back pain usually heals on its own. The body gradually breaks down the protruding disk material and takes it away, relieving the pressure on the nerve. Recovery takes longer than with muscle strain, sometimes several months. But if one is patient, most attacks resolve without surgery.

Ruptured disks can be so severe that they require surgery. If the nerves to the rectum or bladder are affected, causing incontinence, surgery is done right away. Prolonged pain or weakness is another reason for surgery or for other techniques for relieving pressure on the nerve.

Back Pain Emergencies

Some uncommon causes of back pain require medical attention right away. If the vertebra collapses, it can crush the spinal cord, causing paralysis of the legs, which could be permanent. Cancer—especially prostate and breast cancer—that has metastasized to the vertebra can lead to this situation. So can infection of the vertebra. Immobilization and surgery or radiotherapy (or in the case of infection, antibiotics) should be begun as soon as this problem is recognized. Dissecting aneurysm, a tearing of the main artery in the chest and abdomen, also can cause back pain. This pain, which is usually accompanied by other symptoms such as shock, is so severe that patients seek emergency care.

BACK PAIN

Question	To See Clinician If . . .	When
1. Patient's name, age, telephone number		
2. Are you leaking urine?	Yes	2
3. Do you have weakness or numbness in the legs?	Yes	8
4. Have you ever had any kind of cancer?	Yes	8
5. Do you have a fever?	Yes	8
6. Are you alarmed because the pain is so severe?	Yes	8
7. Does the pain run down the back of your leg?	Yes	24-72

EMS = Activate EMS SYSTEM	24-72 = Appointment within 3 days
2 = See ASAP (within 1–2 hours)	72+ = Appointment in 4 days or more
8 = See same day	

High priority items appear in color.

ADVICE

Patients with acute low back pain who do not have reasons for being seen right away (such as incontinence, paralysis, or shock) should be advised to remain at home; they would have difficulty doing almost any kind of work in any case.

- Patients can assume any position and do any activities that are comfortable to them, but should avoid heavy lifting.
- Cold (such as ice cubes in a bag) on the affected area (replaced in a few days by heat) helps relieve symptoms, as do over-the-counter medications such as aspirin or ibuprofen.
- Patients should continue this approach for as long as it takes for the pain to subside, often a few days but sometimes more. They should not rush their return to normal activities but wait until a day after the pain is gone, to avoid relapse.
- **If new symptoms arise, such as weakness or numbness, they should contact the clinician.**

CHAPTER 33

■ ■ ■ ■ ■ ■ ■ ■ ■ ■ ■ ■ ■ ■

Breast Pain in Nursing Mothers

Susan Stangl, MD, MSEd

Although breastfeeding should generally be a natural, painless process, some mothers will experience pain before, during, or after nursing. Often this pain is temporary and resolves as the mother gets used to the process of nursing. Other situations may be more serious and could indicate infection. If a nursing mother complains of breast pain, several things need to be determined:

- What is the location of the pain? Is it in the nipples? The breast itself?
- When does the pain occur? With nursing? At other times?
- Is the breast tender to touch?
- Does the mother have a fever or chills?

> All breastfeeding women who have persistent breast pain of any cause should be observed while nursing and counseled on their technique.

Nipple soreness is probably the most common complaint of breastfeeding women. A woman may have anything from slight discomfort in the nipple at the onset of feeding to severe pain due to cracked nipples. The mild pain that a woman may experience when she first puts the baby on the breast before the milk "lets down" is generally normal and does not require treatment unless it is severe. Perhaps encouraging the mother to trigger the "let down" by massaging her breast before putting the baby on the nipple may help.

Severe nipple pain may result from cracked and irritated nipples and is often caused by poor nursing technique. A variety of measures may be taken to relieve the soreness and help the nipples heal. Rotating nursing positions will keep the baby from sucking repeatedly from the same part of the nipple. Starting with the less sore breast may help, as may short, frequent nursings. Making sure the areola is well back in the baby's mouth so the baby is not sucking just on the tip will also help to avoid soreness. It also is important for the mother to break the suction from the baby's mouth on the nipple before pulling the nipple out.

To help heal cracked nipples, the nipples should be allowed to air dry after each feeding, possibly using a sunlamp (while taking care to avoid burning) or a blow dryer on the cool setting. After air drying, a small amount of nipple cream or bland ointment may be used on the nipples, with care taken not to clog the pores. Rubber breast shields should be avoided and should only be used to help pull out a retracted nipple while feeding. Bra pads, which may stick to the nipples when they dry, should also be avoided. An ice pack may relieve nipple soreness.

Nipple pain may also be caused by thrush, or a yeast infection in the baby's mouth, which shows up as white patches. Older babies may teethe on the breast or bite while nursing.

Breast engorgement may occur if the breasts become overly full because the mother is not nursing often enough. The breasts will feel hard, warm, tender, and full, with shiny skin and often a flat nipple. It will be difficult for the baby to nurse and get the entire areola in his mouth. Warm packs, frequent nursing, and hand-expressing milk before nursing to relieve the engorgement may solve the problem so the baby can latch on properly.

Plugged ducts may occur because of caked secretions within a milk duct. There may be an area of local tenderness within the breast, often accompanied by a tiny lump in the area. Ducts become plugged from going too long between feedings, nursing in the same position all the time, or wearing a too-tight bra that causes pressure under the arm, causing one or more of the milk ducts not to open.

A plugged duct can be treated by nursing more often, starting with the affected breast and using positions that are different from the usual ones. It helps to position the baby's chin closest to the sore spot, as that will give the strongest sucking action. While nursing, massage the area. Moist heat in the form of showers or hot packs may help break up the lump. Avoid using nipple cream, and clean off dried secretions from the nipples. Be sure the bra fits properly.

Mastitis is a breast infection caused by *Staphylococcus aureus* bacteria. The symptoms of mastitis are breast pain, fever, and flulike symptoms such as body aches. It may start with a plugged duct or decreased nursing frequency. Mastitis is most common when a mother is just beginning to nurse, when the mother is breastfeeding less often, or during weaning. It is important for mastitis to be treated promptly so it does not progress to a breast abscess.

> All flulike symptoms in a nursing mother should be considered mastitis until proven otherwise.

The mother should continue nursing, because it is important to empty the breast as much as possible. If the baby is unable to nurse, hand expression or a breast pump may be used. Hot compresses should be placed on the breasts. The mother should go to bed and rest as she would with the flu or any other severe infection. Antibiotics that are active against staph, such as dicloxicillin or cephalexin, should be prescribed. If antibiotics cannot be started right away, the symptoms may be treated for 24 hours with hot packs and frequent breast emptying. If the symptoms persist, antibiotics must be started. Patients with mastitis who receive antibiotics must be followed until the problem resolves.

Breast abscess is a serious infection of the breast that requires surgical drainage. The patient will have fever, chills, and an exquisitely tender area in the breast at the site of the abscess. Abscess is most likely to occur in a patient with mastitis who is weaning her baby.

A
D
U
L
T

BREAST PAIN IN NURSING MOTHERS

Question	To See Clinician If . . .	When
1. Patient's name, age, telephone number	Per clinician preference	
2. Do you have fever or chills?	**Yes**	2
3. Is the breast tender to touch?	Yes	8
4. Are the nipples cracked?	If present for several days and does not respond to usual measures in body of chapter	24-72
5. Do your breasts feel full and hard? (engorged)	If present for several days and does not respond to usual measures in body of chapter	24-72
6. Is the baby having trouble nursing?	If present for several days and does not respond to usual measures in body of chapter	24-72

EMS	= Activate EMS SYSTEM	24-72	= Appointment within 3 days
2	= See ASAP (within 1–2 hours)	72+	= Appointment in 4 days or more
8	= See same day		

High priority items appear in color.

ADVICE

Home Management

- For sore nipples and breast engorgement, suggest short, frequent feedings in a variety of positions. Be sure the areola is all the way in the baby's mouth.
- Allow cracked nipples to dry and avoid skin irritants.
- Plugged ducts require frequent feedings, massage, hot packs, and a properly fitted bra.
- If a patient with suspected mastitis cannot be seen immediately, hot packs and frequent breast emptying (nursing, pumping, or hand expressing) may be started, or the patient may be started on antibiotics over the phone and seen the next day.
- Continue breastfeeding.
- Acetaminophen (Tylenol) may be used for pain relief.

CHAPTER 34

Burns

Ina Cushman, PA-C

Extreme heat injures the skin to varying depths, depending on the length of exposure. Very hot water, a hot radiator, a burner on the stove, fire, and electricity can all cause burns to the skin.

Burn injuries are described by depth of injury. A first-degree burn is an injury to the most superficial layer of skin. It results in redness, warmth, and discomfort, but the skin remains intact. Underlying tissue is not injured. A second-degree burn is a partial-thickness injury to the skin. A partial-thickness burn goes through the epidermis but spares the nerves. It results in blisters, which may or may not be intact; the skin may appear pink to white. A superficial partial-thickness burn will heal by itself, but the most current theories of burn management subscribe to grafting of deep partial-thickness injuries. A deep partial-thickness burn can be very difficult to distinguish from a full-thickness or third-degree burn. A full-thickness burn goes through all layers of skin to fat and destroys nerves. The skin may appear white, black, or charred-looking.

> It may take 48 hours or more before the depth of a burn injury can be accurately determined.

Patients with major burn injuries should be immediately transported via ambulance to a hospital for stabilization and then taken to a burn center. The percentage of the body surface that is burned can be estimated using the "Rule of Nines" (Fig. 34–1). Also, burns around the entire circumference of any body part require transport to the hospital, because they can cause swelling, interruption of blood flow, and tissue ischemia.

Inhalation injury must be ruled out in cases of fire. Electrical injuries can additionally result in cardiac abnormalities, muscle necrosis, fractures, and renal failure. All high-voltage injuries must be seen at a burn center. Burn injury can also occur from chemical exposure; in the home, some cleaning solutions may present this danger.

To triage a burn injury adequately, one must identify the mechanism of the burn, its location and approximate size, the depth of injury to the skin, and additional injuries or illnesses. Identifying the mechanism of injury will suggest whether additional injury may coexist (e.g., inhalation with fire), whether it is a chemical burn, or whether high-voltage electricity was involved (e.g., lightning). You should identify whether areas at high risk were involved (face, hands, feet, or perineum), determine the size of the burn relative to the body's surface area, and get a description of what the burn looks like so you can estimate the depth of the injury.

Identification of burn injury in the elderly, diabetic, or otherwise immunocompromised patient is of major importance. These patients may have compromised wound healing with underlying chronic disease.

Adult

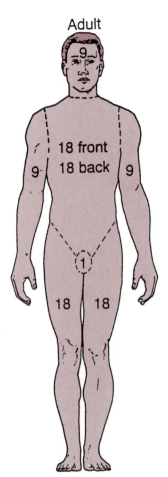

FIGURE 34-1 The Rule of Nines for calculating the body surface area (such as the percentage of surface area burned) in an adult. (From Singer, AJ, et al: Emergency Medicine Pearls, ed. 2. FA Davis, Philadelphia, 2001, p 217, with permission.)

Partial-thickness burns covering less than 15% of the total body surface area and full-thickness burns of less than 2% can be treated in the outpatient setting. These burns need to be seen in the office as soon as possible. Judicious use of oral narcotics may be required to manage pain adequately in the early course of the burn. Even small full-thickness burns need to be evaluated for location. In some areas, early grafting may provide faster healing with less scarring.

BURNS

Question	To See Clinician If . . .	When
1. Patient's name, age, telephone number		
2. Where is the burn?	Face, hands, feet, or perineum.	EMS
3. What kind of burn is it?	Electrical or chemical burn.	EMS
	Burn from fire with inhalation injury.	EMS
4. Describe the burn to me.	Skin is white, black, or charred-looking (third-degree burn) over an area more than the size of your hand.	EMS
	Third-degree burn less than the size of your hand.	2
	Skin is pink to white with blisters (second-degree burn) over an area more than the size of your back.	EMS
	Second-degree burn less than the size of your back.	2
	Skin is red and warm, without blisters (first-degree burn).	2
5. Is your skin clammy, moist, and cool? Do you have palpitations or confusion?	Yes.	EMS
6. When was your last tetanus shot?	More than 10 years ago or do not know.	8
7. Do you have any other medical conditions?	Diabetes mellitus or immunocompromise (including use of corticosteroids [prednisone] or cancer chemotherapy).	2
8. If the burn is not a new event, when did it occur? What made you call now?	More than 2 days ago and signs of infection (cloudy fluid, foul odor), uncontrolled pain, or failure to improve.	8

EMS = Activate EMS SYSTEM	24-72 = Appointment within 3 days
2 = See ASAP (within 1–2 hours)	72+ = Appointment in 4 days or more
8 = See same day	

High priority items appear in color.

ADVICE

- Advise the caller to remove sources of injury if possible. Clothing or other covering that is hot may continue to keep heat in and should be removed.
- If the area is large, a clean sheet wet with cool (not cold), clean water may be used to cover the area until EMS has arrived.
- The patient should be kept warm to prevent shock.
- If the burn area is small (the size of a quarter to a fifty-cent piece) and not over a joint surface, hands, feet, face, ears, or perineum, it should be immersed in cool (not cold), clean water for 20 to 30 minutes, then covered with antibiotic ointment and a dry, sterile dressing.
- Blisters that are intact should be left that way if at all possible. They provide a sterile environment and natural dressing for skin healing to occur. This process can take approximately 5 to 7 days, after which the blister will dry up and peel off, revealing new and somewhat delicate skin underneath.
- The patient should come into the office if the blister fluid appears cloudy or develops a foul odor.
- Pain of outpatient burns may be managed by acetaminophen or ibuprofen in appropriate doses if the patient does not have peptic ulcer disease or an allergy to these medications and is not taking an anticoagulant.
- Avoid friction to the area.
- Avoid sun exposure to burned areas for 1 year to decrease scarring.

A
D
U
L
T

CHAPTER 35

■ ■ ■ ■ ■ ■ ■ ■ ■ ■ ■ ■ ■
■
■
■
■

Chest Pain

William D. Carlson, MD, PhD

Chest pain is a symptom that can be caused by a number of different diseases. Probably the one that is of the most concern to clinicians is **coronary insufficiency,** disruption of the blood flow to the heart muscle, the myocardium. This disorder may have many different symptoms; chest pain is a common and well-known one. How urgent the response needs to be depends on whether the insufficiency is in the form of a **myocardial infarction (MI), unstable angina,** or **stable angina.** To further complicate the situation, there are a number of other causes of chest pain, some of which may necessitate a call to 911 and others of which require less acute treatment. The more common disorders that must be differentiated from coronary insufficiency include:

- Pericarditis
- Aortic dissection
- Pulmonary embolus
- Gastrointestinal diseases
- Musculoskeletal pain

As will be explained, MI, unstable angina, pericarditis with tamponade, aortic dissection, and pulmonary embolus require the immediate attention of skilled medical personal and transportation to an emergency room at a acute care hospital. Other disorders can be treated in the outpatient setting but may require attention within 24 hours.

Determining whether the patient is experiencing an MI (commonly known as a heart attack) is probably the first order and relies on establishing the nature and duration of the pain and its association with other symptoms. MI is the result of the acute blockage ("occlusion") of a coronary artery caused by a platelet-rich clot forming on a plaque within the artery. The occlusion prevents blood from reaching the myocardium and causes cell death and scarring. MI may be preceded by symptoms of chest pain with exertion or at rest. The pain of MI is usually described as being deep inside the middle of the chest and has the character of someone pressing on the patient's chest or a band tightening around the patient's chest. It may radiate to the jaw, throat, teeth, shoulder, back, or arm. It is frequently associated with symptoms of nausea, vomiting, difficulty breathing, feeling warm all over, breaking out in a cold sweat, palpitations, dizziness, or loss of consciousness. The pain of an MI is usually intense but rarely lasts for more than several hours.

Unstable angina is almost as urgent as MI because it frequently indicates that an MI will occur soon and early treatment can prevent the MI and permanent damage to the heart muscle. Unstable angina is a process in which atherosclerotic plaques activate platelets, producing thrombi (blood clots) that narrow the coronary artery and prevent adequate blood flow to the heart muscle. It usually begins with chest pain during exercise, coming on more frequently and with less and less exertion until the pain is occurring at rest. It can have a course of several weeks or days, but occasionally it starts with pain occurring at rest for a period of hours. Stable angina, on the other hand, has a very characteristic pattern in which the pain is consistently associated with the same degree of exertion. The symptoms of nausea, vomiting, dizziness, and shortness of breath, which may accompany MI, are usually absent with both unstable and stable angina.

Pericarditis, inflammation around the heart, is sometimes difficult to differentiate from MI or unstable angina. The inflammation produces fluid between the heart and the membrane that surrounds it. When fluid builds up in this closed space, a condition called **tamponade,** it can prevent the heart from filling with blood, causing low blood pressure and difficulty in breathing. It is important to determine whether a patient reporting chest pain has any symptoms suggesting pericarditis or tamponade. The chest pain associated with pericarditis is usually more severe if the patient is lying down and often is relieved when the patient sits up. It may be worse when the patient takes a deep breath. The pain usually comes on gradually over a period of days, but it can begin more quickly. Associated symptoms such as nausea and dizziness are much less common than with MI.

Aortic dissection is a process in which a channel develops between two layers of the wall of the aorta, the main artery leaving the heart. This channel can measure only a few centimeters, or it can involve long segments of the aorta. It can cause rupture of the aorta or can compromise the blood supply to various regions of the body by blocking any of the arteries that come off the aorta. Dissection usually occurs in patients who have weakened aortic structures and may already have had damage to the aorta. Patients usually experience severe, tearing pain in the chest, radiating to the back.

Pulmonary embolus, blockage of an artery to the lungs by a blood clot, frequently appears as shortness of breath and chest pain associated with taking a deep breath. Usually, however, air hunger and difficulty breathing are features that are more prominent, and these patients are much less likely to have other symptoms such as nausea or dizziness than are patients with MI.

Other disorders that produce chest pain include musculoskeletal pain such as **costochondritis** (inflammation of rib cartilage) or injuries from physical trauma, disorders of the stomach and esophagus, inflammation of the gallbladder, irregular heart rhythms, anxiety, and primary pulmonary hypertension. These disorders usually have other features that are more prominent and lack the associated symptoms of nausea, dizziness, and so on.

Establishing the cause of chest pain symptoms is extremely important because the lives of patients with one of several disorders may be saved by prompt action. It is difficult to provide a single criterion that will establish a diagnosis; often the overall picture is what leads to appropriate action. Pay attention to your gut feeling about any particular patient and realize that you are extremely unlikely to be correct in your diagnosis every time. Because of the difficulty in establishing the diagnosis and the seriousness of the causes, however, it is better to err on the side of more prompt evaluation than on the side of later evaluation. Myocardial infarction, unstable angina, pericarditis with tamponade, aortic dissection, and pulmonary embolus are life-threatening disorders that require immediate attention in an acute hospital. EMTs should be dispatched with haste for any patient you suspect of having any of these problems.

A
D
U
L
T

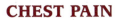

CHEST PAIN

Question	To See Clinician If . . .	When
1. Patient's name, age, telephone number		
2. Is the patient conscious?	No.	EMS
3. Is there pain now?	Yes—Go to question 4. No—Go to question 7.	
4. Is the pain in the middle of the chest and crushing, pressing, or radiating to the arm?	Yes.	EMS
5. Is the pain associated with sweating, difficulty breathing, nausea, or dizziness?	Yes.	EMS
6. Is there a history of coronary artery disease, heart attack (myocardial infarction), or angina?	Yes.	EMS
7. Is there a history of coronary artery disease with angina? If so, is this a change in the pattern of angina?	Yes to both.	EMS
8. Has the pain been occurring at rest or with minimal exertion?	Yes.	EMS
9. Have there been any recent episodes of fainting?	Yes.	EMS
10. Is there shortness of breath?	Yes.	2
11. Is there a history of pulmonary embolus, deep venous thrombosis, or congestive heart failure?	Yes.	2
12. Does nitroglycerin (NTG) relieve the pain?	Yes.	2
13. Does taking a deep breath make the pain worse?	Yes.	2
14. Does moving the arm reproduce the pain?	Yes.	8
15. Does pressing on the chest reproduce the pain?	Yes.	24-72
16. Do antacids relieve the pain?	Yes.	24-72
17. Are there any other symptoms?	Yes.	8
18. Has the chest been injured?	Yes.	8

CHEST PAIN (Continued)

Question	To See Clinician If . . .	When
19. Is there much discomfort?	Yes.	2
	No—Call patient back within 24 hours to follow up.	

EMS = Activate EMS SYSTEM	24-72	= Appointment within 3 days
2 = See ASAP (within 1–2 hours)	72+	= Appointment in 4 days or more
8 = See same day		

High priority items appear in color.

ADVICE

Patients who are thought to be having an MI should be counseled to sit down but not lie down while waiting for emergency medical services to arrive. If aspirin is at hand, they should take one. Patients who have nitroglycerin should place a tablet under their tongue. These patients also can be advised to take several slow, deep breaths. Keeping these patients calm is important, and usually this is most easily accomplished by keeping them focused on simple tasks.

For patients whose symptoms indicate some non–life-threatening problem such as a muscle strain or digestive disorder, see the appropriate chapters for home management advice. The staff member should call back within 24 hours to make sure the patient is OK and arrange any necessary followup.

CHAPTER 36

Colds and Flu

Richard N. Winickoff, MD

Each winter there is a surge in respiratory infections caused by the confinement of the population indoors and the attendant exposure to disease-causing agents spread by microdroplets and from infected hands. For the most part, these respiratory illnesses are mild and self-limited, but they can be more severe. The elderly and those with other chronic diseases are especially susceptible to the complications of flu and other respiratory infections. Separating those patients who require an office or even emergency room visit from those with mild infections is often a difficult challenge.

A variety of microbial organisms, from bacteria to viruses to fungi, produce respiratory infections. Viruses are by far the most common of these, and the most common upper respiratory infection (URI) is the common cold. People have an average of four colds per year, so colds are no stranger to anyone. They often start as a localized sore throat and then progress to a runny, stuffy nose with sneezing. Fever may be present. These symptoms, confined to the nose and throat, define the common cold, or URI. Associated symptoms such as sinus congestion, a dull pain in all the sinuses of the head (above and below the eyes), plugged and stuffed ears with popping, and occasional cough can also occur.

> If more severe symptoms are present in the sinuses, ears, or chest (bronchial tubes), the patient may be suffering from a more severe respiratory infection such as sinusitis, otitis, or bronchitis.

If the pain in a sinus becomes severe and localized, or if there is green or brown drainage from the nose, bacterial sinusitis is likely to be present. Fever is more likely in this case than in an uncomplicated URI. If the ear symptoms move from plugging to pain, and if fever is present as well, the problem is likely to be an ear infection (otitis media). If coughing is severe, especially if green or brown sputum is produced, bronchitis or pneumonia may be present. All of these problems are usually complications of URIs but may occur in the absence of the usual throat and nasal symptoms characteristic of that condition. The importance of diagnosing these complications is that they all respond to antibiotics, unlike URIs, which do not. Telephone questions should be directed at discerning the presence of these complications.

All of these conditions occur in other seasons besides winter, but winter is the peak season for them. In spring and fall, similar nasal symptoms associated with itchy, runny eyes may be the result of allergies, and cough may be due to asthma. In summer, swimmer's ear is more often the cause of an earache than middle ear infection. Yet all of these conditions need to be considered at all times of year.

A word should be said about flu (influenza) and pneumonia, two conditions that definitely increase in the winter. Flu is characterized by fever and muscle aches followed

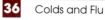

by cough that gets increasingly severe over a few days. It can be debilitating and rarely fatal, especially in those with pre-existing heart or lung disease or other chronic disease, and in the elderly. Flu can progress to pneumonia and in those cases is especially dangerous.

COLDS AND FLU

Question	To See Doctor If . . .	When
1. Patient's name, age, telephone number	Over age 60 and in any distress	8
2. Do you have shortness of breath or chest pain?	Yes	2
3. What is your temperature?	Greater than 103°F	8
	Greater than 101°F but less than 103°F	24-72
4. Do you have any heart or lung disease or other serious medical condition?	Yes	8
5. Do you have bad pain in one of your sinus areas?	Yes	8
6. Are you coughing up bloody sputum?	Yes	8
7. Are you coughing up green or brown sputum?	Yes	8
8. Do you have green or brown drainage from your nose?	Yes	24-72
9. How long have you had a cough? Is it improving?	More than a week, not improving	24-72

EMS	= Activate EMS SYSTEM	24-72	= Appointment within 3 days
2	= See ASAP (within 1–2 hours)	72+	= Appointment in 4 days or more
8	= See same day		

High priority items appear in color.

ADVICE

Patients with the common cold will have predominantly nasal symptoms of sneezing and runny nose. These can be treated with a decongestant-antihistamine cold tablet such as Actifed. Mild sore throat, muscle aches, and low-grade fever that often accompany the common cold are best treated with acetaminophen (Tylenol). If these are the only symptoms, the patient does not need to see the doctor.

If there is a flu epidemic, which is common in the winter, patients should be discouraged from coming to the doctor if they have the typical flu symptoms of aches and pains; fever up to 103°F; weakness; soreness in the throat, larynx, and trachea; and nonproductive cough. The best advice to such patients is to stay in bed and take acetaminophen and lots of fluids.

Patients who have had a cough for less than a week and who have no chest pain or fever can treat the symptom with a guaifenesin (gweye-uh-FEN-eh-sin) syrup like Robitussin or a "house brand" product with the same ingredients (with or without dextromethorphan). Dextromethorphan (a cough suppressant) is helpful if the cough is very bothersome and is interfering with sleep. Even if the cough has lasted more than a week, the patient can use the same syrup if the cough is improving and he or she has no fever and is not producing green, brown, or bloody sputum.

Patients with sinus congestion can take an antihistamine-decongestant such as Actifed or Dimetapp or use a decongestant nasal spray such as Afrin, twice daily for up to 3 days. Use for longer than 3 days leads to rebound blockage of nasal passages when the medication wears off. Inhaling steam from a shower or bowl of hot soup often helps as well.

Patients over the age of 65 and those with chronic diseases, especially heart and lung diseases, should be encouraged to receive the pneumococcal vaccine when they are better, to protect against the most common type of bacterial pneumonia in the future. These people should also be advised to get a flu shot every year, because many of the serious lung infections occur during flu epidemics. Both of these vaccines are highly effective.

A
D
U
L
T

CHAPTER 37

■ ■ ■ ■ ■ ■ ■ ■ ■ ■ ■ ■
■
■
■
■
Constipation

Deborah J. Wald, MD

When patients call complaining of constipation, it is important to determine what they mean by this term. Although many people believe it is necessary to have a bowel movement every day, in fact normal stool patterns can range from three stools a day to one every 3 days. People with normal stool frequency may also use the term to describe straining or pain with defecation or small, hard stools. Constipation is a very common complaint, and in adults its incidence increases with age.

Most constipation does not require urgent treatment. It is important to be aware, however, of three serious medical problems that can present as constipation:

- **Bowel obstruction** can be caused by malignancy, stricture (narrowing) of the bowel, adhesions (internal scarring) from past surgery, or volvulus (twisting of a loop of bowel). If obstruction is complete, patients usually have severe, cramping abdominal pain, nausea and vomiting, and may not be able to pass either gas or stool per rectum. Complete obstruction is a medical emergency.

- **Nerve dysfunction** causes constipation when there is decreased sensation in the anal/rectal area or poor function of smooth muscle or voluntary sphincters. Acute constipation in a patient with back pain (due to injury or metastatic cancer) may indicate spinal cord compromise and requires immediate evaluation or imaging of the spine to prevent further loss of function. Patients with altered sensory or sphincter function from underlying health problems such as multiple sclerosis, spinal cord injury, or diabetic peripheral or autonomic neuropathy are at higher risk of chronic constipation and fecal impaction.

- **Fecal impaction** is a collection in the rectum of hardened stool, which the patient is unable to expel. This complication of chronic constipation is more common in the elderly or debilitated patient. Patients may be incontinent of liquid stool, which seeps around the impaction. Treatment often requires manual disimpaction, followed by a careful bowel regimen to avoid recurrence.

In patients with nonurgent constipation, several factors in the history can help direct treatment:

- **Diet:** Inadequate fiber intake leads to small, hard stools that may be difficult to evacuate. High-calcium foods such as cheese may also be constipating, and inadequate fluid intake contributes to constipation.

- **Drugs:** Many prescription and over-the-counter drugs cause constipation. In evaluating constipation of recent onset, ask about any change in dose or medication. Most notorious are opioids and calcium channel blockers, but many common drugs, including aluminum-containing antacids, NSAIDs such as ibuprofen, and any medicine with anticholinergic side effects (e.g., antihistamines, some antidepressants, and some drugs taken for urinary incontinence) can also cause constipation.

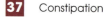

- **Laxative abuse:** People who chronically use stimulant laxatives develop tolerance, requiring higher doses to have the same effect, and they often become dependent on laxatives to move their bowels. Other agents are safer for chronic use.

> Nonmedicinal treatment recommendations, as discussed in the Advice section at the end of this chapter, are safe for virtually any patient. Recommendations for medications, on the other hand, may need to be tailored to the patient's other medical problems and the severity of the constipation. In most cases, it will be appropriate to consult with the clinician for specific telephone advice before recommending even over-the-counter medication for constipation.

A
D
U
L
T

CONSTIPATION

Question	To See Clinician If . . .	When
1. Patient's name, age, telephone number		
2. When was your last stool?	More than 1 week ago.	8
3. What have you tried already to relieve the constipation?	This is second phone call for same problem, symptoms are worsening, or patient requests appointment.	8
4. Do you have any other symptoms?	• Nausea, vomiting, severe abdominal pain, no gas or stool per rectum. • Severe back pain *and* recent back injury or history of cancer.	EMS
5. Do you have any other medical problems?	• Patient is frail, bedridden, or has neurologic impairment (stroke, MS, dementia, etc.). • Other major medical problems. (Consult with clinician for specific telephone advice or whether more urgent visit is required.)	8 24-72

EMS	= Activate EMS SYSTEM	24-72	= Appointment within 3 days
2	= See ASAP (within 1–2 hours)	72+	= Appointment in 4 days or more
8	= See same day		

High priority items appear in color.

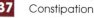

ADVICE

Patients should call back if their symptoms are not relieved within 24 to 48 hours or at any time if they develop increased abdominal pain, nausea or vomiting, or other urgent symptoms.

Nonmedicinal Recommendations

Nonmedicinal recommendations are appropriate for any patient with constipation:

- **Increasing fiber** in the diet produces larger, softer stools, which are easier to expel. Fruits, raw vegetables, whole-grain foods, bran, popcorn, potato skins, and peanuts are high in fiber. Patients who find it difficult to get the recommended 10 to 30 grams of fiber per day from their diet alone can use fiber supplements (bulk agents) such as psyllium.
- **Increasing fluid intake** and getting **regular exercise** also help relieve and prevent constipation.
- Taking advantage of the **gastrocolic reflex** can make it easier to move the bowels. A full stomach stimulates the sigmoid colon and rectum to empty. Because of diurnal rhythms, this impulse may be stronger in the morning. Patients should sit on the toilet and try to defecate for 5 to 10 minutes after breakfast and perhaps again after supper. They should avoid straining for more than 5 to 10 seconds at a time.

Medications

Most medications for constipation are available without a prescription, but the clinician should be consulted to ensure that specific recommendations are appropriate for the severity of the constipation and the patient's underlying medical problems.

- **Bulk agents,** or fiber supplements such as Metamucil or Citrucel, are safe for long-term use. These often cause bloating initially but are well tolerated if patients start with a low dose and advance gradually. Fiber supplements are only effective if taken with sufficient fluids. They should be avoided by patients with mechanical obstruction or strictures.
- **Osmotic agents** increase the water content of the stool. Docusate is safe for long-term use but has a very weak effect. Magnesium salts, such as milk of magnesia or magnesium citrate, are safe for most patients but should not be used by patients with renal failure. Poorly absorbed sugars such as lactulose or sorbitol may cause bloating but are safe for long-term use and are very effective in chronic constipation. Mineral oil is **not** recommended, because it can cause lipid pneumonia in patients at risk for aspiration, and it may decrease the bioavailability of fat-soluble vitamins.
- **Stimulant laxatives** are best avoided, because the colon becomes dependent on them with time. Many "natural" or "herbal" laxatives fall within this category, and are **not** safe to use chronically. Oral stimulant laxatives include senna, aloe, cascara, rhubarb, phenolphthalein, and bisacodyl. They are likely to cause cramping, because they stimulate intestinal muscle activity. Bisacodyl, of course, is a stimulant agent whether you give it orally or rectally (see Suppositories, below), and neither type is recommended for chronic use. The oral form is more likely to cause cramping.
- **Suppositories and enemas** function by causing local irritation or rectal distension, or by directly stimulating sigmoid and rectal motility. They include hypertonic phosphate enemas (Fleet's enemas) and bisacodyl and glycerin suppositories. These are safe even in severe constipation because they work to empty the colon "from below." They are useful in relieving constipation acutely but generally are not recommended for chronic use. Patients with renal failure should not use phosphate enemas. Bisacodyl suppositories do have a role in the treatment of severe constipation but should not be used chronically.

CHAPTER 38

■ ■ ■ ■ ■ ■ ■ ■ ■ ■ ■ ■
■
■
Cough
■

John D. Goodson, MD

Most adult patients will accept a moderate amount of coughing. Calls for assistance, advice, or evaluation generally come when the cough is so severe that it interferes with the usual life routine, when the cough is associated with other significant complaints or symptoms, or when the cough has lingered for an extended period.

Although coughing represents a normal physiologic process, it can also develop as a consequence of any irritation in the respiratory tract. In some cases, the irritation can be secondary to a more serious condition elsewhere, such as cardiac decompensation or gastroesophageal reflux. As a symptom, cough should be taken seriously; the clinical evaluation should proceed until an explanation is identified or the cough has fully resolved.

> The telephone evaluation of cough should focus on the nature, duration, and severity of the cough and other associated complaints or symptoms.

When evaluating the nature of a cough, the goal is to determine how much the cough interferes with usual activities and whether the cough has responded to simple over-the-counter remedies, such as cough drops or lozenges. Generally, the evaluation of chronic cough should be timely, but not urgent. Patients with acute persistent cough, especially those whose sleep has been significantly disturbed (interrupted sleep or the inability to get to sleep due to cough) should be evaluated soon or managed over the telephone in a fashion that allows patient reassessment if needed.

Cough with sputum production suggests a more acute inflammatory process, usually an infection (e.g., pneumonia, bronchitis) or asthma. Cough with blood (hemoptysis) is frightening to the patient, but in most cases the blood represents more serious inflammation, not a malignancy. It is helpful to hear the patient cough over the telephone. The presence of audible wheezing suggests acute bronchospasm (asthma). Cough in this situation may require active bronchodilator therapy.

When evaluating the other symptoms or conditions associated with cough, it is most critical to focus on infection, bronchospasm (asthma), and cardiovascular decompensation. Infectious causes include sinusitis, bronchitis, and pneumonia. Asthma (see Chapter 61, Wheezing) should always be considered, remembering that the causes of airway irritation can be infectious, chemical (including direct chemical irritants such as gastroesophageal reflux), drug-related (e.g., ACE inhibitors), or allergenic. If the patient is known to have other concurrent conditions, these should be identified. They may include heart disease, lung conditions, or any factors that would predispose the patient to infection, such as advanced age or immune system compromise.

> If the patient has a chronic medical condition, review the record or discuss it with the primary clinician to determine whether cough is a recurrent presenting complaint of that illness.

The patient's prior experience with cough and its management is helpful because the cough may represent an exacerbation of a known illness. When cough is a recurrent symptom, the patient can generally help to establish the pace and urgency of evaluation.

Treatment for cough should focus first on any underlying condition, especially any infections, as well as pulmonary or cardiac disease. In the absence of more serious conditions, cough can be managed for a short period of time (1 to 3 days) with empiric over-the-counter medications. The patient and provider should agree on the goals for this treatment and specific symptoms, such as worsening cough at night or fever, that would require an earlier call-back if they arise.

A
D
U
L
T

COUGH

Question	To See Clinician If . . .	When
1. Patient's name, age, telephone number		
2. Do you feel short of breath?	Severely (having difficulty talking).	EMS
3. Are you wheezing?	Yes—See Chapter 61, Wheezing.	
4. Do you have a fever?	Very high (above 102.5°F).	2
	High (101.6°F to 102.4°F) or moderate (100.0°F to 101.5°F).	8
	Low-grade (below 100°F).	24-72
5. How long has the cough been present?	Acute (less than 48 hours).	8
	Moderately acute (2 to 14 days).	24-72
	Chronic (more than 2 weeks).	72+
6. How often do you cough?	Frequently (once or more per hour).	8
	Moderately often (several times a day).	24-72
	Occasionally (once or twice a day).	72+
7. Does the cough keep you up at night?	Frequently (every night).	8
	Moderately often (a few nights).	24-72
8. Are you raising phlegm or sputum?	Yes, bloody or yellow, green, or brown.	8
9. Do you have chest pain or tightness?	Yes—See Chapter 35, Chest Pain.	
10. Do you have other medical conditions (e.g., HIV or AIDS, asthma, congestive heart failure, coronary artery disease, sinusitis, rhinitis)?	Yes.	8

**SEE CHAPTERS 61, WHEEZING; 35, CHEST PAIN;
OR 36, COLDS AND FLU, AS APPROPRIATE.**

EMS = Activate EMS SYSTEM	**24-72** = Appointment within 3 days	
2 = See ASAP (within 1–2 hours)	**72+** = Appointment in 4 days or more	
8 = See same day		

High priority items appear in color.

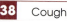

ADVICE

Patients with cough should be instructed to try an over-the-counter (OTC) cough suppressant unless it is medically contraindicated. Those that are most effective, such as Robitussin DM, contain dextromethorphan. Some OTC cough suppressants contain a significant amount of alcohol; these should be avoided.

- Persistent cough can physically exhaust patients. The patient should be instructed to call back for a prescription cough medicine (usually one containing codeine) if the OTC suppressant does not control the cough within 12 hours.
- All patients should try to avoid environmental factors, such as smoke or cold and dry air, that will irritate the lung and worsen cough.
- All patients should try to maintain hydration by drinking one or two extra glasses of water per day, unless medically contraindicated.
- Patients using inhaled drugs should be asked if their inhalers could be empty. Empty canisters will float when placed in a bowl of water.
- Goals of treatment, such as significant improvement or disappearance of the cough within a specific period of time (e.g., 24 to 48 hours), should be agreed upon. If at the end of this time, the goal has not been reached, the patient should call back. Patients should also call back if the cough worsens, fever develops, or the phlegm increases in amount or deepens in color to yellow, green, or blood-tinged.
- The patient should be instructed to call back immediately if shortness of breath develops. The situation should then be reviewed with the clinician.

CHAPTER 39

■■■■■■■■■■■■■

Diarrhea

Jeannette M. Shorey, MD

Diarrhea is an increase in the fluid volume and frequency of stools. Although many people refer to any change in their usual bowel habits as diarrhea, most authorities agree with defining diarrhea to mean more than three liquid stools per day.

Acute Diarrhea

> Acute diarrheal illnesses usually are caused by infections with viruses, bacteria, or parasites. Most episodes of this very common problem are self-limited and mild, lasting 2 to 4 days. A history of recent travel to tropical or third world countries or recent exposure to other people with diarrhea provides helpful clues to infectious causes.

A common, noninfectious source of acute diarrhea is "food poisoning," which is caused by toxins produced by bacteria that have contaminated food. Some of these toxins cause vomiting as well as diarrhea. The vomiting or diarrhea typically begins 6 to 12 hours after ingesting the contaminated food.

Other important noninfectious causes of acute diarrhea include drugs (e.g., laxatives, magnesium-containing antacids, colchicine, quinidine, and antibiotics used within the past 3 months), inflammatory bowel disease, fecal impaction, and ischemic colitis. The latter two causes typically occur in elderly people.

> Brisk bleeding from any portion of the gastrointestinal track can be life-threatening, and initially stools may look like "ordinary diarrhea" before they become frankly bloody.

Telephone staff must ask about the following key features of an acute diarrheal illness when determining the urgency of a patient's evaluation:

- The presence of blood in the diarrhea.
- Fever greater than 101°F.
- Severe abdominal pain.
- Evidence of dehydration (e.g., lightheadedness, fainting, severe weakness, malaise) and inability to take in oral fluids.
- Other illnesses (e.g., immunosuppressing illnesses like diabetes, cancer, or AIDS).
- The patient's age (frail elders tolerate diarrhea far less well than young, generally healthy adults).

Patients who meet these criteria must be advised to seek evaluation by a clinician. The evaluation should be considered an emergency if the patient feels faint or clammy, is in severe pain, is passing visible blood in the stool, or was frail at baseline.

Chronic Diarrhea

Chronic diarrhea is usually defined as more than three very soft or watery stools per day, lasting for more than 3 weeks. It can trouble patients for weeks, months, or even years. It may be a functional symptom (irritable bowel syndrome); a manifestation of a food intolerance (e.g., lactose intolerance or gluten intolerance); or evidence of a chronic parasitic infection, inflammatory bowel disease, malabsorption caused by chronic pancreatitis, one of several diseases of the small intestine, endocrine disorders, secretory colonic polyps, or intestinal infections associated with HIV or AIDS.

When a patient's call concerns chronic diarrhea, telephone staff must determine if there is a new, acute problem atop the chronic problem. As with all calls about chronic problems, the staff must genuinely consider the answer to the question: "Why is this patient calling about this now?"

DIARRHEA

Question	To See Clinician If . . .	When
1. Patient's name, age, telephone number		
2. How long have you been having diarrhea?	Less than 3 weeks: Go to question 3. More than 3 weeks: Go to question 15.	
3. Have you fainted in association with the diarrhea?	Yes.	EMS
4. Are the stools maroon, repeatedly bloody, or accompanied by significant amounts of bright red blood (estimated at ¼ cup or more with a single stool)?	Yes.	EMS
5. Are the stools black or tarry?	Yes.	2
6. Do you feel lightheaded with changes of position and at risk of fainting?	Yes.	2
7. Can you take in and keep down significant quantities of fluids?	No.	2
8. Do you have severe, constant abdominal pain along with the diarrhea?	Yes.	2
9. Do you have a fever higher than 101°F?	Yes.	8
10. Do you have an immunosuppressive disease (e.g., HIV/AIDS, leukemia, lymphoma) or take immunosuppressive drugs (e.g., chemotherapy for any cancer, antirejection drugs after any organ transplant, prednisone at doses greater than 10 mg/day)?	Yes.	8
11. Are you elderly or weak? Do you have diabetes mellitus or coronary artery disease?	Yes.	8
12. Is the diarrhea associated with intermittent, crampy pain?	Yes.	24-72
13. Have you recently traveled to a third world country or been exposed to other people with a similar diarrhea?	Yes.	72+
14. Are you taking any medications known to cause diarrhea (e.g., laxatives containing magnesium; colchicine, quinidine, antibiotics in the last 3 months)?	Yes. Advise discontinuing the medication and contacting the primary care provider for a possible office evaluation.	72+

A
D
U
L
T

157

DIARRHEA (Continued)

Question	To See Clinician If . . .	When
15. If the diarrhea has been present for more than 3 weeks, has it worsened in the past few days?	No.	72+

EMS = Activate EMS SYSTEM		24-72 = Appointment within 3 days
2 = See ASAP (within 1–2 hours)		72+ = Appointment in 4 days or more
8 = See same day		

High priority items appear in color.

ADVICE

Patients with diarrhea who have none of the key features that point to the need for prompt evaluation can be advised to do the following:

- Rehydrate or maintain normal body fluid volume with frequent, small amounts of clear liquids containing salt and sugar (e.g., broth, Gatorade, Jell-O, popsicles, dilute apple juice, flat soda).
- Avoid milk products, all fruit juices (except clear), coffee, alcohol, fatty or fried foods, and high-fiber foods until the diarrhea has resolved.
- Gradually increase to small amounts of simple foods such as boiled rice, applesauce, baked potatoes, dry toast, and crackers, eating several small meals throughout the day rather than three large ones, until the diarrhea resolves.
- Call the primary care provider if the diarrhea has not resolved in 48 to 72 hours.

Over-the-counter medications such as Imodium, Pepto-Bismol, and Kaopectate work by different mechanisms to slow the frequency of diarrhea. If the patient is sick enough to warrant prompt evaluation by a clinician, these should not be recommended. If the patient is generally healthy at baseline, however, and has no fever and no evidence of dehydration or blood in the diarrhea, any one of these preparations can be used, following the package directions.

CHAPTER 40

Ear Pain

Richard N. Winickoff, MD

Earache is not as common in adults as in children, but it is a frequent occurrence nonetheless. It occurs in two major settings: (1) as a complication of colds or hay fever and (2) as a consequence of water getting into the ear.

In the case of colds or hay fever, the upper airway passages are swollen and inflamed, causing the eustachian tubes between the ear and the upper part of the throat to close.

> When the eustachian tubes are shut, normal secretions from the lining of the middle ear cannot drain out. Bacteria that reside throughout the upper airway passages start to multiply within the trapped fluid. The result is a bacterial infection of the middle ear called acute otitis media.

If the fluid builds up but there is no inflammation, the condition is called otitis media with effusion (formerly, serous otitis media). Otitis media with effusion is likely to cause ear plugging and decreased hearing rather than pain. It may also occur after an airplane ride.

When water gets into the external ear canal, it can disrupt the skin and allow bacteria or even fungi to grow there. A condition may develop called external otitis, or swimmer's ear. Like otitis media, it can either be very painful or not, depending on the amount of associated inflammation. Both conditions may cause a plugged feeling and decreased hearing.

Another condition that can cause a plugged feeling in the ear is accumulated ear wax. It may be painful if it is packed tightly, especially if the patient has pushed it in further with a cotton swab.

EAR PAIN

Question	To See Doctor If . . .	When
1. Patient's name, age, telephone number	Per physician's preference	
2. Is the ear painful?	Yes	8
3. Is temperature above 100°F?	Yes	8
4. Is the external ear canal swollen?	Yes	8
5. Is there plugging, clicking, or decreased hearing?	Yes	24-72
6. Have you been swimming in the past week?	Yes	24-72
7. Did the symptoms start after an airplane flight?	Yes	24-72

EMS	= Activate EMS SYSTEM	24-72	= Appointment within 3 days
2	= See ASAP (within 1–2 hours)	72+	= Appointment in 4 days or more
8	= See same day		

High priority items appear in color.

ADVICE

Pain or Fever

If the patient has pain or fever, he or she will need either to be seen and evaluated before therapy is started or to speak with the physician about interim therapy. Acetaminophen (1000 mg up to four times a day) should be recommended until the patient can be seen.

If the patient has been swimming recently, it is best to recommend an office visit to make a definitive diagnosis. At the office visit, the clinician can decide if the infection looks bacterial or fungal and can prescribe appropriate therapy based on the examination.

Plugging, Clicking, Decreased Hearing

If the symptoms are limited to plugging, clicking, or decreased hearing, ask if the patient has been swimming recently or has flown in an airplane. It may be possible to resolve blocked eustachian tubes (e.g., from air travel) with simple over-the-counter decongestants such as pseudoephedrine (Sudafed), 30 to 60 mg every 4 to 6 hours. As noted above, if the patient has been swimming, recommend an office visit.

Patients who get ear blockage or pain regularly during air travel can take up to 120 mg of pseudoephedrine 30 minutes before takeoff. Studies show a 50% reduction in the incidence of such symptoms when this treatment is used.

If the patient is susceptible to ear wax buildup, it would be appropriate to arrange an ear irrigation, not necessarily involving the physician. An interim measure in such cases is glycerin-peroxide ear drops. Two drops should be inserted in the affected ear nightly, and the patient should lie with the affected ear up for 2 minutes after application. This procedure frequently loosens and occasionally may remove the wax. After a few days, the patient may use a soft-bulb ear syringe to remove loosened wax.

ADULT

CHAPTER 41

■ ■ ■ ■ ■ ■ ■ ■ ■ ■ ■ ■ ■
■
■
■
■
Eye Pain and Foreign Bodies

Richard S. Weinhaus, MD

Patients frequently call about problems involving one or both of their eyes. The chief complaint may be pain in or around the eye, a foreign-body sensation, or a disturbance of vision. The challenge in the phone encounter is to determine whether the problem is serious or minor and to determine whether the patient needs to be seen, and if so, how urgently. Visual disturbances are discussed in Chapter 59.

An Approach to Eye Pain

Obviously, new-onset or severe pain requires more urgent attention than chronic or mild pain. In taking the phone history, it is important to try to pinpoint the location of the pain. If it becomes clear that the pain is not coming from the eye itself, but from the temple, for instance, the diagnoses being considered will of course be different.

Even if patients cannot precisely localize their pain, they are frequently able to differentiate a deep pain, suggesting a problem in or behind the eye, from a foreign-body type of pain, suggesting a problem with the ocular surface. In the latter case, the eye is frequently described as feeling scratchy, gritty, dry, or as if "something is in the eye." (See the section later in this chapter on Foreign Bodies and Foreign Body Sensation.)

> If the patient volunteers that the painful eye also has decreased vision or pain on exposure to bright light (photophobia), this is a red flag that a serious problem may be present.

Be aware, however, that patients with migraine headaches, which are common and almost always benign, may also report the need to withdraw from brightly lit or noisy environments.

Pain Behind the Eye (Orbital Pain)

Pain in virtually any of the structures surrounding the eye can localize so that patients may describe the pain as being "in the eye" or "behind the eye" in the same way that patients with cardiac ischemia may experience pain involving their left arm or shoulder. Thus migraine or tension headaches, sinus inflammation, and dental, nasal, or frontal pain may all localize to the region around the eye. Typically, the patient states that the eye aches or feels sore. The pain is frequently described in the same way as other headache pain, as being deep, dull, aching, persistent, throbbing, recurrent, and so forth (see Chapter 45, Headache). Frequently the pain will involve both eyes or a larger area than the eye itself.

> If a patient with orbital pain complains of double vision, forward bulging of the eye (proptosis), or pain on extremes of gaze, beware of a serious problem.

Brief, intermittent, knifelike pains behind the eye, with intervals of no discomfort, are a common complaint and are not serious.

Eyelid Problems Causing Pain

The most common cause of lid pain is a **stye,** a localized, painful, tender mass near the margin of the eyelid. Styes are usually caused by staphylococcus bacteria and are similar to pimples. A stye is not usually a severe problem. The mainstay of treatment is warm compresses to get the pus within the stye to drain. In addition, most patients will be happier if treated with a topical antibiotic such as erythromycin ointment.

Whether a patient needs to be seen for a stye or can be managed by phone depends on the patient's level of pain and anxiety and on whether a more widespread bacterial infection may exist. Widespread cellulitis of the lid (also called preseptal cellulitis or periorbital cellulitis) is extremely painful and tender, like cellulitis involving other portions of the face. It is an urgent medical condition.

If a patient reports the new onset of severe pain, tenderness, redness, and swelling in the area of the lower lid toward the nose, an acute infection of the tear drainage system (dacryocystitis) should also be considered. It is also an urgent medical condition.

The main entity to be distinguished from cellulitis of the lid is an allergic swelling of the lids. Within minutes of onset, the swelling can become so severe that one or both lids totally close. Unlike cellulitis, however, the lids are not tender or painful. Intense itching is usually present. Sometimes patients report exposure to an inciting agent such as pollen or animal hair. Cold compresses and oral antihistamines are the mainstays of treatment.

A contact dermatitis of the lids may also be confused with cellulitis. Usually the patient has recently used a topical antibiotic. Neomycin is a notorious offender and gentamicin is also frequently implicated, but almost any eye drop or ointment (including erythromycin ointment) can be the cause. The caller will describe the lids as being red, leathery, and uncomfortable but not severely painful.

Iritis and Other Causes of Intraocular Pain

Iritis

"Intraocular" means inside the eye. Intraocular inflammation is called **iritis,** inflammation involving the iris and surrounding structures. A spontaneous complaint of eye pain made worse by exposure to light (photophobia) strongly suggests iritis. The patient usually reports that the eye is red and tender. Vision may or may not be decreased.

Iritis is relatively common. It can begin on its own or it can be the result of other eye problems such as trauma, a corneal ulcer, or angle closure glaucoma. If severe, it can lead to permanent visual loss. Iritis is usually treated with topical steroids, which should be prescribed by an ophthalmologist.

Iritis needs to be evaluated and treated. If you suspect iritis, arrange to have the patient seen by an ophthalmologist, both to assess its severity and to rule out other conditions that may have caused it. For example, a bacterial corneal ulcer may cause severe iritis, but in this case, the eye needs to be treated with intensive antibiotic drops and not with steroid drops. Starting such a patient on steroid drops can be disastrous.

Acute Glaucoma (Acute Elevation in Intraocular Pressure)

An acute rise in intraocular pressure for any reason will lead to eye pain and nausea. (In contrast, **chronically** elevated eye pressure, such as is seen in chronic open angle glaucoma, does not typically cause pain or a sensation of pressure.) With an acute rise in intraocular pressure, the eye is frequently red and tender. If the eye pressure is high enough, the patient will also have swelling (edema) of the cornea, leading to a complaint of generalized fogginess and rainbow-colored halos around lights. Acute angle closure glaucoma is a rare condition that presents with this constellation of symptoms. It is more likely to occur in older patients. An attack can occur spontaneously or can be precipitated by anything that causes the pupil to dilate, including dilating drops, drugs with anticholinergic effects, and some over-the-counter cold medicines. It is an ophthalmic emergency.

Do not confuse the symptoms of an acute rise in intraocular pressure, which is rare (except in postoperative patients), with those of a visual migraine, which is common. Both conditions can cause pain, nausea, visual disturbance, and photophobia, but the visual disturbance in migraine is described as being shimmering, wavy, jagged, shifting in position, and so forth. Furthermore, the visual disturbance in migraine typically lasts only 10 to 30 minutes, whereas the fogginess seen with acutely elevated intraocular pressure lasts until the pressure is reduced.

Postoperative Patients

Patients who have recently had cataract or other intraocular surgery frequently call after hours. If their chief complaint is pain, decreased vision, photophobia, or nausea, they should be referred immediately to their ophthalmologist. In contrast, mild postoperative discomfort or a mild foreign body sensation is not usually an urgent problem. All postoperative patients should be advised, however, that if their symptoms are getting worse, they may have an urgent problem.

Foreign Bodies and Foreign Body Sensation

Patients frequently call because of a foreign body or foreign body sensation in the eye. The goal of the telephone encounter is to determine whether the patient needs to be seen and how urgently.

Nearly all of the foreign bodies reported by phone are superficial. They are small airborne particles of metal, sand, or other debris that blow or fall into the eye and become embedded on the front surface of the eye or the inside surface of the upper lid. The onset is unmistakable.

The phone calls are frequently from mechanics or from others exposed to dust or wind. The patient reports that "there is something in my eye" or "up under my lid." Vision is usually normal but may be blurry owing to increased tearing because of the irritation. (Vision will also be decreased if the foreign body has lodged in the central part of the cornea.) The patient may report that blinking makes the eye feel worse and that keeping the lid closed makes it feel better. The level of discomfort may range from minimal to extreme.

Unless the patient has experienced serious trauma or has been struck by a high-velocity projectile such as a fragment from metal striking metal while hammering or grinding, there is little concern that the foreign body has actually penetrated the eye.

Foreign bodies are best managed by an ophthalmologist. If none is available, these patients may be treated by an emergency room physician with experience using a slit

A
D
U
L
T

lamp. If the call comes at night and the patient is reasonably comfortable, he or she may be seen the following morning.

A corneal abrasion (a scrape on the front surface of the cornea) can cause the same symptoms as a corneal foreign body, but patients with corneal abrasions may be evaluated and managed by their primary care physician. Usually their history will distinguish between the two. Common causes of corneal abrasions include a scratch from paper, a fingernail, an eyeliner brush, or the branch of a plant. Vision will be decreased if the abrasion involves the central portion of the cornea or if there is increased tearing due to irritation.

Foreign body **sensation** is one of the most common chief complaints of patients calling by phone. In addition to actual foreign bodies and corneal abrasions, any condition that causes inflammation, drying, or infection of the surface of the eye can cause a foreign body sensation. Usually the patient cannot pinpoint the exact time of onset. Some conditions, such as a corneal ulcer or a herpes simplex corneal infection, are serious and require urgent attention. Other common conditions, including dry eye, conjunctivitis, and a turned-in eyelash (trichiasis), usually are not serious or urgent.

Because so many conditions can result in foreign body sensation, it is seldom possible (or necessary) to make a diagnosis by phone. The important thing is to be able to identify conditions that may lead to permanent visual loss and to arrange for these patients to be seen urgently.

> If a foreign body sensation is associated with eye pain, decreased vision, or pain on exposure to light (photophobia), this is a red flag that a sight-threatening problem may be present.

On the other hand, if there is ocular **discomfort** rather than pain, if vision is not decreased, and if there is no photophobia, it is much less likely that the problem is sight-threatening.

Foreign Body Sensation in Contact Lens Wearers

Be especially wary of the combination of severe pain and foreign body sensation in a contact lens wearer. This combination has two main causes. One is a bacterial corneal ulcer, a serious condition requiring urgent treatment with topical antibiotics. Patients who **routinely** sleep with extended-wear contacts in place are at especially great risk for corneal ulcers. Typically, the pain and redness get worse even hours after the contact lens has been removed.

The second cause is overwearing syndrome. The eye becomes red and painful because of drying and lack of oxygen. Typically, the symptoms get worse the longer the contact lens is worn and improve within hours after the contact lens has been removed. Daily-wear contact lens patients who forget to remove their contact lenses on a particular night may awake in the morning with a severe overwearing syndrome. If, on the other hand, they have occasionally slept with their contacts in place before without problems, suspect a corneal ulcer.

EYE PAIN AND FOREIGN BODIES

Question	To See Clinician If . . .	When
1. Patient's name, age, telephone number		
2. How long has the problem been present?		
3. Is the eye or eyelid very painful?	Yes—the eye. Yes—the eyelid.	2 8
4. In addition to the pain, has the vision decreased?	Yes.	8
5. Does the eye hurt if you look at a bright light?	Yes.	8
6. Did something *suddenly* get into your eye?	Yes.	8
• If so, were you hammering, grinding, or using power tools?	Yes.	2
7. Have you had this problem before?	No, new onset or serious recurrent problem. (Urgency depends on history and symptoms.)	
8. Are you using prescription eye drops or ointments?	Yes, but worse anyway. (See eye specialist. Urgency depends on history and symptoms.)	
9. Do you have any serious medical problems?	Yes. (Urgency depends on history and symptoms.)	
10. Do you wear contact lenses? If so, is the eye painful?	Yes.	8
11. Have you had recent eye surgery? If so, do you have severe pain, decreased vision, or nausea?	Yes.	2

SEE ALSO CHAPTER 59, VISUAL DISTURBANCE.

EMS = Activate EMS SYSTEM	24-72 = Appointment within 3 days
2 = See ASAP (within 1–2 hours)	72+ = Appointment in 4 days or more
8 = See same day	

High priority items appear in color.

A
D
U
L
T

ADVICE

Styes

If the problem sounds like a small stye, advise warm compresses with a warm washcloth (which has been placed under the hot water tap). It should be rewarmed each time it cools, for a total soak time of 10 minutes, three times a day. A prescription for a topical antibiotic ointment can be obtained from the physician.

Iritis

Sometimes patients with a long history of iritis will call at night to report a flare-up and to ask if it is all right to restart their topical steroid drops. If the diagnosis is certain, and the patient can be seen by or speak with the ophthalmologist in the morning, it is reasonable to advise restarting the steroid drops in the interim. No one other than an ophthalmologist should prescribe steroid drops by phone.

Foreign Body or Foreign Body Sensation

For minor foreign body sensation, over-the-counter artificial tears, ocular lubricating ointment, or both may provide substantial relief.

Retained Contact Lens

Sometimes a patient who wears contact lenses will call with the concern that they cannot find a contact lens and they do not know whether it fell out or "got stuck behind the eye." Reassure these patients that although a contact lens can become lodged under the upper lid, it cannot migrate to a dangerous location. If there is no pain or foreign body sensation, the lens has probably fallen out and the patient does not need to be seen unless anxious.

CHAPTER 42

Fainting

Robert H. Fletcher, MD, MSc

Fainting (the specific name is **syncope** [SIN-ko-pee]) is the sudden loss of consciousness with recovery within minutes. Syncope is common. Many people experience an attack at some time in their life. Many attacks are not brought to medical attention.

Syncope is caused by transient loss of blood flow to the brain, usually when the blood pressure falls below a certain level. All causes of syncope have in common a failure to get enough blood to the part of the brain that maintains consciousness. Without the nutrients in blood, especially oxygen, unconsciousness ensues within seconds.

Syncope can occur without warning or can be preceded by nausea, sweating, pallor, warmth, and a feeling that one is going to pass out. In the usual course of events, a patient with syncope will begin to recover consciousness within a minute or two, be fully alert (although perhaps groggy) in 5 minutes, and have no after-affects other than perhaps fatigue, anxiety, and sluggishness for several hours.

The severity of syncope can vary. At one extreme, an attack may not go all the way to unconsciousness, a situation called "near-syncope." At the other extreme, a patient with a cardiac event that initially appears to be syncope may not recover, a situation that has been called "irreversible syncope."

> Although usually harmless, syncope can be dangerous in two ways. One is straightforward: the patient can be injured by falling during the attack. The other is the possibility that syncope has been caused by an abnormal heart rhythm that could lead to sudden cardiac death if it recurs and is more severe the next time.

Is It Syncope?

Syncope should be distinguished from other forms of sudden altered consciousness or dizziness that have other causes:

- **Vertigo** is a sensation of movement; patients feel as if the room is spinning or they are spinning in the room. Patients do not feel as if they are going to pass out. With severe attacks, nausea and vomiting can occur, just as in motion sickness. Vertigo is caused by diseases of the inner ear, the part that senses position, and its connections to the brain.
- **Seizures** are often accompanied by rhythmic muscle contractions. If the patient loses consciousness, it usually takes at least a half-hour to recover. Sometimes there are warning symptoms such as hallucinations, called an "aura." Seizures are caused by abnormal electrical activity in the brain.
- **Dizziness.** Some patients, especially those who are elderly or anxious, complain of frequent attacks of a difficult-to-describe feeling of weakness and unsteadiness.

Often the exact reason for these attacks is not discovered, but panic attacks are one cause.

- **Low blood sugar,** especially in diabetics who take insulin, can cause unconsciousness, but usually the symptoms come on gradually.

Kinds of Syncope

A common form of fainting is **postural syncope**—fainting when standing up suddenly from a sitting or lying position, or fainting after prolonged standing, especially in the heat. The elderly often have a fall in blood pressure when they stand up. If the drop is severe, it can lead to fainting. Pregnant women also have a tendency to faint when they are on their feet for a long time. Dehydration (from excess sweating, vomiting, or diarrhea) predisposes to postural syncope.

Vasovagal syncope is passing out when in a state of fear or anxiety (for example, after bad news or in a dental chair). The cause is a sudden failure of blood pressure regulation, influenced by both the pumping of the heart and the tone of the blood vessels.

Cardiac syncope is less common but more dangerous. This type of syncope is caused by a transient cessation of heartbeat. It is difficult to know whether this is the cause in any one patient; there are no characteristic symptoms. But there are clues: older age, already having heart disease, recurrent attacks, and the absence of the characteristic situation and symptoms that suggest postural or vasovagal syncope.

Transient ischemic attacks (TIAs) occur when the brain's circulation is obstructed, causing that part of the brain to malfunction, after which the obstruction is rapidly relieved. TIAs are similar to strokes except that they clear up completely within 24 hours (by definition) and often within minutes, leaving no neurologic deficit such as weakness, numbness, or difficulty thinking. But during most attacks there are specific neurologic symptoms. Syncope alone is an uncommon way for TIAs to occur.

Straining to cough or urinate also can bring on an attack of fainting.

Syncope is often the result of a combination of causes. For example, a soldier may faint during inspection after prolonged standing in the hot sun, especially if he or she had diarrhea the night before. The cause of an attack of this sort may be obvious after a few simple questions. It may be so obvious to the patient that he or she does not even seek medical care.

Evaluation

The causes of syncope are usually evident after careful questioning and a simple examination. Sometimes testing, such as wearing a monitor to detect abnormal heart rhythm, is necessary. Sometimes the causes of a single attack are not known for sure, despite testing.

Whatever the cause of syncope, the patient may be injured, especially if he or she was standing when it happened, by falling and striking hard objects such as table corners or the floor. If the patient becomes unconscious while caught in an upright position (for example, when sitting in a chair), the body's attempt to recover blood pressure by getting horizontal is thwarted and the brain may be without oxygen long enough to cause some seizure activity. This is alarming to witnesses, and to the patient if he or she is told about it, but it does not necessarily mean that the patient has a seizure disorder.

Telephone questions should be directed toward three issues:
1. Was the attack syncope or another kind of spell?
2. Was the patient injured during the attack?
3. Might the heart have been responsible for the attack?

A
D
U
L
T

FAINTING

Question	To See Clinician If . . .	When
1. Patient's name, age, telephone number		
2. How long was the patient unconscious?	Still unconscious	EMS
	Several minutes	2
	A few minutes	8
3. Did the patient have other symptoms during or after the attack?	Yes, chest pain	EMS
	Yes, numbness and weakness	2
	Yes, muscle jerking	2
4. Was the patient injured during the attack?	Yes, struck head, can't stand up, or bleeding	2
5. Does the patient have a heart condition or previous stroke?	Yes	2
6. Has the patient had similar attacks before?	Yes	8
7. Was there an obvious reason for fainting?	Yes, (just got bad news, for example)	24-72
8. Is the patient or family and friends worried about the attack?	Yes, very upset	8

EMS = Activate EMS SYSTEM

2 = See ASAP (within 1–2 hours)

8 = See same day

24-72 = Appointment within 3 days

72+ = Appointment in 4 days or more

High priority items appear in color.

ADVICE

In most cases fainting is harmless. It happens because of a temporary fall in blood pressure, so that the brain does not get enough oxygen. After an attack, patients may feel unusually tired but should otherwise feel as they normally do. But some precautions are worthwhile for several hours after the attack:

- Take it easy in calm surroundings.
- Drink lots of fluids.
- Get up very slowly to allow the body to adjust to the standing position.
- Do not try to do anything complicated or dangerous right away.

Fainting does not necessarily indicate a serious disease or cause permanent damage. Patients may need to be treated for injuries incurred if they fall during an attack.

If the patient is elderly or is known to have heart disease, or if the patient faints repeatedly, he or she should be examined by the clinician. Someone who saw the incident should accompany the patient to help describe what occurred.

ADULT

CHAPTER 43

Fever

Juliet K. Mavromatis, MD ▪ *William T. Branch, Jr., MD*

Fever is a physiologic response to infection or inflammation that occurs when the hypothalamus of the brain increases the body's thermal set point. In contrast, hyperthermia results when the body's cooling mechanisms fail—it is nonphysiologic. Fever is a symptom of many medical conditions ranging from benign to life-threatening. It is generally defined as an oral temperature greater than 98.6°F, or 37°C. However, in normal people temperature may fluctuate throughout the day, ranging from 97.0°F (36.1°C) to 99.3°F (37.4°C).

When an adult patient calls complaining of fever, it is critical to differentiate among conditions requiring various degrees of medical intervention. Unlike children, who generally have few if any underlying medical conditions, many adults have underlying medical problems that complicate triage, making it challenging to propose general guidelines that may be used for each individual.

The most common cause of a fever is infection. Infections may be viral, bacterial, fungal, or parasitic. Medical conditions such as immunodeficiency caused by chemotherapy, malignancy, chronic steroid use, splenectomy, or infection with human immunodeficiency virus (HIV) provide clues about what types of infections a patient might have. Certainly these conditions increase the risk of serious infections that require more rapid medical intervention. In addition, certain diseases make patients more susceptible to particular infections. Examples include:

- Renal failure (arteriovenous shunt infections, bacteremia)
- Diabetes (cellulitis, osteomyelitis)
- Chronic obstructive pulmonary disease (COPD) (bronchitis, pneumonia)
- Sickle cell anemia (cholecystitis, pneumonia)
- Alzheimer's disease (urinary tract infections, pneumonia, decubitus ulcers)
- Liver disease (spontaneous bacterial peritonitis)

Noninfectious conditions also cause fever. Drug fever may result from a multitude of medications ranging from antibiotics to seizure medications. Often such medications also produce a rash. Other conditions that should be considered are:

- Malignancy (e.g., lymphoma)
- Connective tissue disorders (e.g., rheumatoid arthritis)
- Overactive thyroid gland
- Inflammatory states (e.g., sarcoidosis, pulmonary embolus, deep venous thrombosis, and pericarditis)

Generally fever is not harmful to patients, but there are exceptions. Fever increases cardiac demand and so may worsen symptoms in patients with congestive heart failure or coronary artery disease. In demented patients and the elderly, fever may cause worsening of mental status. In these cases, and in most cases in which fever is greater than 104°F, antipyretic medications should be used.

FEVER

Question	To See Clinician If . . .	When
1. Patient's name, age, telephone number		
2. What is your temperature?	Higher than 103°F.	8
3. How long have you had fever?	More than 72 hours.	8
4. Do you have any other serious or chronic medical conditions?	Asthma, renal failure, congestive heart failure, COPD, diabetes, cancer, AIDS, dementia, sickle cell anemia, coronary artery disease.	8
5. Do you have other symptoms?	None.	24-72
• Throat problems?	Inability to swallow own secretions.	EMS
• Fainting?	Yes.	EMS
• Chest pains?	Yes, not affected by breathing.	EMS
	Yes, breathing causes pain.	2
• Shortness of breath?	Yes, severe.	EMS
	Yes, mild.	8
• Delirium?	Yes.	EMS
• Headache with stiff neck, avoidance of light?	Yes.	2
• Abdominal pain?	Yes, severe.	2
	Yes, mild.	8
• Diarrhea, nausea, vomiting?	Yes, and not able to drink.	2
	Yes, able to drink.	8
• Urinary problems?	Pain or difficulty in urinating, urinary frequency, back pain.	8
• Skin problems?	Swollen or tender red skin, rash.	8
• Cough?	Productive cough.	8
	Cough with ear, nose, or throat symptoms.	24-72
• Ear, nose, or throat symptoms?	Nasal congestion, sneezing, sore throat, painful glands, ear pain.	24-72
• Joint or muscle ache, swollen joints?	Yes.	24-72
6. Have you recently been in contact with someone else who is sick?	Yes.	24-72

EMS	= Activate EMS SYSTEM	24-72	= Appointment within 3 days
2	= See ASAP (within 1–2 hours)	72+	= Appointment in 4 days or more
8	= See same day		

High priority items appear in color.

A
D
U
L
T

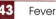

ADVICE

Patients with no underlying medical conditions who have fever with mild upper respiratory or gastrointestinal complaints can sometimes be managed without an office visit, particularly if they have had contact with someone with a similar illness.

- These patients should be instructed to call back if their symptoms worsen or if the fever lasts more than 3 days.
- Fever-lowering medications include acetaminophen and aspirin. These should be recommended for patients with heart disease or dementia, and for those with fever greater than 104°F, to prevent the harmful effects of fever itself. For others, medication may be administered in the following dosages to relieve muscle aches, chills, sweats, and headache:
  - Acetaminophen (Tylenol), 325 to 650 mg orally every 4 to 6 hours, not to exceed 3 g (about 6 extra-strength or 9 regular tablets or capsules) in 24 hours. People with liver disease should avoid acetaminophen, and those who drink alcohol should take less.
  - Aspirin, 1 to 2 tablets every 4 to 6 hours (for adults only). People with kidney disease or a history of gastrointestinal bleeding should avoid aspirin.
- Treating upper respiratory symptoms with over-the-counter decongestants may be beneficial.
- Nausea, vomiting, and diarrhea may be treated with antiemetics such as compazine and phenergan and antidiarrheal agents such as Imodium, at the clinician's discretion.
- Patients with fever should increase their fluid intake. Solid food is not as important.

Patients who have underlying medical conditions are more complex. The clinician should usually be asked to review the individual case before the urgency of the visit is determined. Patients who are in nursing homes or have the services of a visiting nurse can sometimes be managed more conservatively with good supervision and follow-up phone calls.

- Patients who have started a new medication within the past week may have drug fever—particularly if there are no other symptoms except perhaps a rash. Pending review by a physician, sometimes a visit may not be necessary.

A
D
U
L
T

CHAPTER 44

Frostbite

Ina Cushman, PA-C

Prolonged exposure to cold causes damage to the skin that is similar to a burn from exposure to heat. Freezing of tissue (frostbite) occurs when skin temperature is around 14°F to 25°F. (Fahrenheit is the scale patients are familiar with.) Environmental factors such as high winds and the moisture content of the air may change the incidence of cold injuries. Other factors such as malnutrition, trauma, immobility of the patient during exposure, and preexisting occlusive arterial disease may add to the incidence of cold injuries. Prevention is key and is achieved by wearing layers of dry clothing and covering all exposed body parts.

> Patients with frostbite should also be evaluated for possible systemic hypothermia, defined as core temperature less than 95°F. Oral thermometers are often not accurate. Rectal temperatures are needed for accuracy in mild cases of hypothermia. Symptoms can include weakness, fatigue, and lethargy. Absence of shivering is a sign of more serious hypothermia. It is important to keep victims warm and dry and to transport them to the nearest emergency room via EMS.

Frostbite is divided into four classes that are similar to those used for burns. Freezing of tissue without blistering heralds first-degree frostbite. Such tissue is gray or white, firm or hard to the touch, feels cool when touched, and often is insensate (cold produces anesthesia). Owing to this anesthesia, symptoms of itching pain and paresthesias (tingling) may not occur until thawing begins. Freezing of tissue with clear blistering heralds second-degree frostbite. Third-degree frostbite involves subsequent death of skin, injury to subcutaneous tissues, and some hemorrhagic blisters. In fourth-degree frostbite, there is full-thickness skin death and involvement of subcutaneous tissues including bone. It often results in loss of the body part or severe deformity. As depth of frostbite increases the depth of injury, there is a decreased range of motion and increased swelling of the body part involved. As thawing occurs, anesthetic effects are lost. Pain increases; the patient notes itching, tingling, and burning pain. Tissue becomes discolored and sometimes gangrenous.

Fortunately, most frostbite patients suffer only mild, superficial frostbite of the extremities. Many can be managed with simple rewarming after removal of outer clothing such as gloves or boots. Affected areas should be rewarmed by applying constant warmth without rubbing. Friction can increase skin injury. Fingers can be placed in the armpits to warm to body temperature. Feet should be dried gently and covered with warm, dry socks. These areas should be protected from undue friction or trauma, and patients should be warned to guard them from further exposure throughout the rest of the cold season.

Rewarming of full-thickness frostbite should only be undertaken if there is no chance of refreezing, which would increase tissue damage and necrosis. Rapid rewarming at temperatures slightly above body temperature has been shown to decrease tissue death. This can be done by immersion of the body part in warm water (about 104°F) for 20 to 30 minutes. Moist heat is preferable, because the temperature is easier to control. Do not attempt to increase temperature by rubbing or exercise. Do not rub the frozen part with snow. The frostbitten areas should remain covered with a sterile dressing, protected from infection and friction. Blisters should remain intact if possible.

Patients with full-thickness frostbite should be evaluated at an emergency room. Extensive superficial frostbite may need hospital observation as rewarming occurs.

Chilblain is a cold injury suffered by many athletes such as skiers, skaters, and climbers. It is a result of chronic exposure to cold, moist air without adequate protection to body parts. Superficial ulcers develop on exposed areas, often face or hands. These areas should be treated with rapid rewarming, protection from trauma, observation for infection, and avoidance of further exposure.

FROSTBITE

Question	To See Clinician If . . .	When
1. Patient's name, age, telephone number		
2. Do you feel sluggish, weak, or fatigued (signs of systemic hypothermia)?	Yes	EMS
3. Describe the frostbitten area.	Gray or white, firm, cool skin with blistering, decreased range of motion, swelling.	EMS
	Gray or white, firm, cool skin. No blistering.	2
4. Are the ears or nose involved?	Yes	2
5. Do you have any other medical conditions?	Diabetes mellitus or immunocompromise (including use of corticosteroids [prednisone] or cancer chemotherapy)	2

EMS = Activate EMS SYSTEM
2 = See ASAP (within 1–2 hours)
8 = See same day

24-72 = Appointment within 3 days
72+ = Appointment in 4 days or more

High priority items appear in color.

ADVICE

- Advise the caller to remove wet clothing.
- If the patient is lethargic, weak, or fatigued, he or she may be suffering from low body temperature. Wrap in blankets and call EMS for transport to the hospital.
- Advise the caller to rewarm the body part quickly if there is no chance of refreezing. Hands with mild frostbite can be warmed by placing them in the armpits or in warm water (about 104°F).
- Advise the caller not to rub affected parts with anything, especially snow. Keep blisters intact if possible.
- Alcohol should not be used on frostbitten skin.
- If frostbite is mild, advise the caller to keep the affected areas clean, dry, and warm. Protect them from friction. Watch for signs of infection.
- Pain can be treated with acetaminophen (Tylenol) or ibuprofen if not contraindicated by peptic ulcer disease, allergy, or anticoagulants.

ADULT

CHAPTER 45

Headache

William J. Mullally, MD

Headache is the most common pain experienced by humans and is the leading complaint for which patients present to a physician. In the United States, 70% of the population will experience a headache in any given year and 1% of office visits are primarily for headaches. For the patient, the headache itself is a disease. For the health care provider, the headache is either an isolated disorder or an element of a more widespread disease. Recurrent headaches are usually benign, but they may signal the presence of a serious underlying disease process such as meningitis, brain tumor, or intracranial hemorrhage. When patients present to a physician with the complaint of headache, they are concerned not only with achieving pain relief but also with being reassured that they do not have a brain tumor.

Classification of Headaches

With a complaint of headache, as with any other medical problem, placing it in a diagnostic category helps one to know whether further testing is needed and suggests treatment approaches. There are four main categories of headaches: migraine, tension-type, cluster, and traction and inflammatory headaches.

Migraine Headaches

A migraine headache is often described as a "sick headache." The pain is usually described as pressure or throbbing and is often accompanied by nausea and vomiting. It is aggravated by light, noise, odors, and movement, so patients may seek a dark, quiet room to achieve pain relief. Most migraine headaches are on only one side, but 30 to 40% affect both sides. Two-thirds of migraine patients also have neck pain. Mood disturbances such as depression, euphoria, irritability, and anger also are quite common in association with migraine, and patients may crave sleep or experience frequent urination or diarrhea before or during an attack. About 20 to 30% of migraine attacks are preceded or accompanied by an "aura"—neurologic symptoms such as blind spots, flashing lights, numbness, or weakness on one side. Such symptoms usually abate by the time the headache appears, but they may persist. The pain of a migraine headache may last from hours to days. Migraine headaches usually begin in the second or third decade of life, and 70% of these patients report a family history of such attacks. The disorder affects about 18 to 20% of women but only 7 to 10% of men. Migraine frequently accompanies menstruation in women.

Tension-Type Headaches

Almost everyone has experienced a tension-type headache at some time. It is usually described as a dull, bandlike sensation or tightness involving the entire head, accompanied by discomfort on both sides of the neck. Elements that accompany a migraine, such as nausea, avoidance of light, and neurologic symptoms, do not occur with a tension-type headache. Some people have infrequent tension-type headaches, but others have persistent pain that can last for days, months, or years. This type of headache is often related to stress, and chronic ones are usually associated with depression. Many patients experience both migraine and tension-type headaches; in fact, tension-type headaches and migraines are components of the same headache continuum.

Cluster Headaches

Patients afflicted with cluster headaches experience one to several headaches per day for 3 to 6 weeks and then remain headache-free for a significant period, commonly 9 to 12 months. The pain of cluster headache is more intense than the pain of migraine but lasts for a shorter time, typically between 5 minutes and 4 hours. These headaches almost always are centered in and around one eye and often are described as a constant, severe pain, as if "a hot poker is being pushed into the eye." The headache often awakens these patients 1 to 2 hours after they go to sleep. Unlike patients with migraine attacks, those with cluster headache will pace the floor rather than remain motionless. Nausea and vomiting are uncommon. Most sufferers do experience tearing from the affected eye and nasal congestion or discharge on that side of the head. Occasionally cluster headaches become chronic, without periods of remission. They affect less than 1% of the population, of whom 80 to 90% are men.

Traction and Inflammatory Headaches

Traction and inflammatory headaches are caused by organic diseases of the skull or its contents. Pain is the result of traction (pulling) or inflammation of the pain-sensitive structures of the cranial vault. Causes include tumors, meningitis, and subarachnoid hemorrhage, as well as less serious disorders such as sinus infection, eye strain, and reduced pressure following a lumbar puncture. Headaches in this category are uncommon.

Diagnosis of a Headache

A detailed patient history and neurologic and physical examination by the clinician is essential to the correct diagnosis of a headache. Atypical headache patterns may suggest that some serious process is underlying the symptom of headache.

A telephone history cannot provide a definitive diagnosis, but it can yield clues. The most important task in telephone triage is to differentiate benign headache patterns from headaches with features that suggest a possible serious underlying disorder requiring immediate care. Such causes for concern include reports of:

- The first or worst headache of the patient's life, especially if it is associated with neurologic symptoms
- A headache that becomes progressively worse over days or weeks
- Headache associated with fever, nausea, and vomiting that cannot be explained by another illness
- Headaches associated with changes in consciousness or difficulty in reading, writing, or thinking
- A headache that does not fit any of the usual patterns or causes

A
D
U
L
T

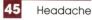
Studies of patients presenting to an emergency room with a chief complaint of headache have found that 25 to 55% have migraine and tension-type headache and 30 to 40% have either an infection or an illness pertaining to the whole body. Fewer than 5% have a serious neurologic condition such as meningitis, tumor, or brain hemorrhage.

HEADACHE

Question	To See Clinician If . . .	When
1. Patient's name, age, telephone number		
2. How severe is the pain? Did it begin suddenly?	Extreme pain (worst of life), beginning suddenly.	EMS
3. Do you have a stiff neck and a fever?	Yes.	2
4. Was there recent head trauma?	Yes.	8
5. Do you have weakness, tingling, numbness, double vision or visual loss, dizziness, inability to speak, mental changes, or loss of consciousness?	Yes to any.	8
6. Are you diabetic? If so, are there symptoms of hypoglycemia?	Yes.	8
7. Do you have nausea, vomiting, tearing from the eyes, nasal congestion or discharge?	Yes to any.	8
8. Do you have an illness such as lupus, AIDS, or immune deficiency?	Yes.	24-72
9. Do you have fever, rash, night sweats, unintended weight loss?	Yes.	24-72
10. Did the headache follow exercise or sexual intercourse? If so, has this happened before?	Yes, and this is the first time. Yes, and this has happened before.	8 24-72
11. Is the location or pattern of this headache different from past headaches?	Yes.	24-72
12. Have you recently consumed alcohol or drugs? Have you just started taking a new medication?	Yes.	24-72
13. (For a woman of childbearing age) What was the date of your last menstrual period? Are you pregnant?	Pregnant or last period more than 4 weeks ago.	8 (blood test) 24-72 (evaluate)
14. Have you been sleepless or fatigued?	Yes.	72+
15. Do you have symptoms of depression, such as weight loss, lethargy, sleep disturbances?	Yes.	72+ 8 (if suicidal)

A
D
U
L
T

HEADACHE (Continued)

Question	To See Clinician If . . .	When
16. Do you get this kind of headache regularly? If so,		
• At what age did they start?	After 50 years old.	24-72
• Describe the usual pattern (onset, severity, character, duration, frequency)	Headaches fit pattern of one of the major types.	72+
• Do certain symptoms usually precede the headache, such as mood change, change in appetite, or visual symptoms?	Yes.	72+
• Is there a family history of similar headaches?	Yes.	72+

EMS = Activate EMS SYSTEM		24-72 = Appointment within 3 days	
2 = See ASAP (within 1–2 hours)		72+ = Appointment in 4 days or more	
8 = See same day			

High priority items appear in color.

ADVICE

Patients who call to complain of headache should be seen for evaluation, with the urgency of that visit depending on their answers. Unless they are already being actively treated for a chronic headache disorder, treatment cannot be prescribed over the telephone. Those who are under active treatment can be advised to continue the treatment program that has been established, with an elective follow-up visit later.

Those whose headaches seem to follow a pattern but who are not being actively treated should be encouraged to keep a log of their headaches and schedule an appointment.

A
D
U
L
T

CHAPTER 46

Head Injury

Marie-Eileen Onieal, MMHS, RN, CPNP

The head is one of the most commonly injured sites of the body. Motor vehicle accidents contribute to 50 to 70% of all head injuries. Other causes are falls, blunt and penetrating trauma, and athletic trauma. In all head injuries, the organ of concern is the brain. Thus, it is of paramount importance in all head injuries for the provider to decide the necessity of hospitalization and consultation with a neurosurgeon. Very few incidents require this level of care, but careful evaluation and follow-up are essential to optimal outcomes in these injuries.

The spectrum of head injuries is wide, ranging from subtle injuries to gunshot wounds. Most head injuries are of the nonpenetrating, closed injury type. It is not uncommon for the injured person to report "seeing stars" after experiencing a blow to the head. The most common injury is a concussion. A concussion is often associated with a loss of consciousness. A longer period of loss of consciousness indicates a more serious concussion. Often, the major symptoms of a concussion are a temporary loss of vision, pallor, listlessness, memory loss, or vomiting. These symptoms can be transitory or last for hours.

The more severe head injuries are brain contusions and hematomas. With these injuries, the brain is bruised or there is frank bleeding into the brain. Associated with these injuries is a disturbance of mental status, partial paralysis, unequal pupil size, or an alteration in vital signs. Other parts of the body may also be injured, and these patients require an immediate assessment for appropriate emergency care.

The history of the injury is key to determining the need for evaluation and treatment. Many patients are dazed or may have lost consciousness following the injury. Others may have been under the influence of alcohol or other mind-altering substances at the time of injury. This impairs the ability to obtain information about the injury. It may be necessary to speak with others who can supply information about the circumstances surrounding the incident.

> A common complaint is a fall with a subtle blow to the head. If the fall is significant, such as from a considerable height, the best course of action is to bring the person in for evaluation. Initially, the patient may complain of headache and nausea, look pale, or experience vomiting. In the hours following the injury, the patient should be closely observed for any worsening of symptoms or change in mental status.

If the fall is insignificant and the person is acting fine, without symptoms of concussion, it is appropriate to explain what signs and symptoms are to be expected and what to watch for at home. The caller should call back if any significant changes occur. Persons who live alone or who are elderly should have someone with them for 24 hours after the injury.

CHAPTER 48

Menstrual Pain

Susan Stangl, MD, MSEd

Menstrual pain (**dysmenorrhea**) may be confined to the pelvic region or may radiate to the hips, lower back, or thighs. Some women with dysmenorrhea also experience nausea, diarrhea, constipation, and headaches. **Primary dysmenorrhea** is menstrual cramping in patients who have no organic disease. It usually begins 1 to 2 years after menarche and often improves by the mid-20s or after the first pregnancy. **Secondary dysmenorrhea** is accompanied by specific conditions such as endometriosis, uterine fibroids, ovarian cysts, pelvic inflammatory disease, adenomyosis, or the use of an intrauterine contraceptive device (IUD).

Because menstrual cramps and their accompanying gastrointestinal symptoms are caused by the release of prostaglandins, the most common effective remedies for menstrual pain are the nonsteroidal anti-inflammatory drugs (NSAIDs), which block the release of prostaglandins. Several of these drugs, including ibuprofen and naproxen, are available over the counter. Aspirin, a mild prostaglandin inhibitor, may also be effective, as may acetaminophen (Tylenol), which does not inhibit prostaglandins but does relieve pain. Sometimes it is necessary to start the NSAIDs before the onset of menstruation to inhibit prostaglandin release and prevent dysmenorrhea. Because prostaglandin levels in the uterus are different for each woman, patients will vary in their response to antiprostaglandin therapy. On occasion, a patient with severe dysmenorrhea that is unresponsive to NSAIDs may benefit from a trial of oral contraceptive pills. Rarely, a patient may be given muscle relaxants or narcotics for severe pain.

Other ways to relieve menstrual pain include taking a warm bath, applying a heating pad to the abdomen, getting in the knee-chest position, or having an orgasm. Exercise and relieving constipation may help. Dietary supplements that may offer some relief include calcium, magnesium, vitamin B_6, and vitamin E. Amphetamines and over-the-counter diet aids may worsen menstrual cramps.

Any patient who does not respond to a reasonable dose of an NSAID (400 to 800 mg of ibuprofen every 6 hours or 275 mg of naproxen every 8 to 12 hours) should be examined to rule out other pathology that may be contributing to her pain.

> If there is a chance the patient may be pregnant, she should be seen to rule out a miscarriage or an ectopic pregnancy.

If the patient has a fever and an infection is suspected, she should be seen immediately. Otherwise, menstrual pain is not an emergency and should be evaluated in the course of a patient's regular gynecologic care, depending on her level of discomfort and the persistence of her symptoms.

MENSTRUAL PAIN

Question	To See Clinician If . . .	When
1. Patient's name, age, telephone number		
2. Is there any chance you could be pregnant?	Yes.	2
3. Do you have a fever?	Yes.	8
4. What remedies have you already tried? Have they helped?	NSAIDs (such as ibuprofen or naproxen); they have not helped.	24-72

EMS = Activate EMS SYSTEM	24-72	= Appointment within 3 days
2 = See ASAP (within 1–2 hours)	72+	= Appointment in 4 days or more
8 = See same day		

High priority items appear in color.

ADVICE

Patients with no symptoms requiring an office visit should be advised to try one or more of the following remedies:

- Take a warm bath or apply a heating pad to the abdomen.
- Try exercising or getting in knee-chest position.
- Take calcium or magnesium supplements.
- Take an NSAID (ibuprofen, 400 to 800 mg every 6 hours, or naproxen, 275 mg every 8 to 12 hours).

A
D
U
L
T

CHAPTER 49

■ ■ ■ ■ ■ ■ ■ ■ ■ ■ ■ ■

Neck Pain

John D. Goodson, MD

Neck pain most commonly is the consequence of an acute injury or neuromuscular irritation from chronic misuse.

> When injury is the cause, rapid assessment is necessary to be certain that the neck is stable and that the patient does not face the risk of permanent neurologic damage to the spinal cord.

The patient with an injured neck needs to be seen by a clinician to establish baseline neurologic and muscular function. Radiologic studies may be indicated. For the patient without a history of injury, the evaluation must proceed quickly but generally not with urgency.

Pain in the neck can arise from a variety of neurologic and musculoskeletal conditions. With trauma, pain reflects either bone fracture, a change in the position of the soft tissue structures of the neck (such as the discs in the cervical spine), or swelling around the joints or nerve roots of the neck. Because the cervical spinal cord is critical in the support of breathing (the high cervical spinal nerve roots supply the diaphragm), any traumatic injury carries some risk of dire outcome. Fortunately, such cervical injuries are rare and are usually identified immediately. Nonetheless, it is possible for neck injury to create an unstable situation wherein the function of the cervical spinal cord is at high risk from any subsequent trauma, however minor.

The cervical nerve roots radiate out from the cervical spinal cord, each supplying a different area of the neck and shoulder. Irritation or injury to these nerve roots can produce pain in the area of nerve distribution, called referred pain. Patients with neck pain will occasionally report referral of the pain to the shoulder, upper arm, or even the fingers.

Though rarely as worrisome as pain from acute injury, neck pain from chronic misuse of the neck can be quite disconcerting to the patient. Many daily activities, such as cradling the telephone by bending the neck to the side or looking repetitively upward by extending the neck, can irritate the soft tissue structures that support the neck. This irritation can produce either local inflammation in the joints and ligaments of the neck or irritation of the nerves supplying the muscles of the neck, which causes muscle spasm. Like traumatic injuries affecting the nerve roots, chronic neck misuse can produce symptoms that extend to the shoulder, arm, and fingers.

Other medical conditions can also produce pain in the neck. These include migraine and tension headache syndromes, anxiety, and others.

The treatment of neck pain begins with an assessment of neck stability. When trauma has preceded the pain, it may be necessary to stabilize the neck with a collar or other device. Even when there has been no trauma, the stability of neck structures must be considered. Elderly patients are especially prone to degeneration of the joints and supporting soft tissues, which may allow structures to slip or change position enough that there is risk of spinal cord injury.

Once stability is assured, patients are provided with pain relief, anti-inflammatory medication, and muscle relaxation, either with heat or medication. Other treatment modalities, such as massage therapy or acupuncture, may be helpful. Physical therapy is generally not started until neck pain has subsided.

Symptoms of neck pain frequently recur unless the tissues are allowed to heal to the maximum extent possible and the patient is prudent in daily activities, avoiding the neck twisting, bending, and extension that tends to cause the greatest stress on neck structures. Patients with recurrent neck pain have generally tried some sort of self-treatment with limited success or know what prescription treatment has worked in the past. This information should be recorded.

NECK PAIN

Question	To See Clinician If . . .	When
1. Patient's name, age, telephone number		
2. Has there been any neck injury or trauma?	Acute trauma (less than 24 hours)	2
	Recent trauma (2 to 14 days)	8
	Remote trauma (more than 2 weeks)	24-72
3. How severe is your neck pain?	Severe (unable to move neck without pain)	8
	Moderate (able to move neck, pain only at the extremes of motion)	24-72
4. Does the pain spread or radiate to other parts of the body?	Shoulders, arms, or fingers	2
	Neck only	8
	Up and down spine	8
5. Do you have any weakness in your shoulders or arms?	Yes	2
6. How long have you had neck pain?	Acute (less than 2 days)	8
	Recent (2 to 14 days)	8
	Chronic (more than 2 weeks)	24-72

EMS = Activate EMS SYSTEM	24-72	= Appointment within 3 days
2 = See ASAP (within 1–2 hours)	72+	= Appointment in 4 days or more
8 = See same day		

High priority items appear in color.

ADVICE

Because of the need to be certain of neck stability, patients with neck pain resulting from an accident or injury should be evaluated by a clinician. Elderly patients may be at higher risk due to underlying joint disease. Patients who also have symptoms such as numbness, weakness, or tingling of the arm or fingers should be discussed with the clinician to determine how the evaluation should proceed.

Some patients with neck pain can be managed without an office visit:

- Instruct patients to avoid positions that put the neck under stress, such as hyperextension (looking above eye level), or excessively twisting and bending the neck (such as cradling a phone).
- Apply heat to the neck to reduce muscle spasms caused by nerve irritation or joint inflammation. Gel-packs that can be heated in a microwave are inexpensive and convenient.
- Control pain with acetaminophen (Tylenol), 325 to 650 mg orally every 4 to 6 hours, not to exceed 3 grams (6 extra-strength 500-mg tablets or 9 regular-strength 325-mg tablets) in a 24-hour period. Older patients and those with liver disease or excessive alcohol consumption should use less. Another drug for pain relief is ibuprofen (Advil, Motrin), 200 to 400 mg every 6 to 8 hours. Patients with ulcer disease, indigestion, or reflux should use these medications cautiously.
- Neck pain frequently can be aggravated during sleep. Using a neck pillow to reduce neck movement during the night may be helpful. Several different types are available.

CHAPTER 50

Nosebleed

Laurence J. Ronan, MD

Nosebleed (**epistaxis**) is an uncommon telephone complaint for adults. Patients call when bleeding is brisk, recurrent, or unstoppable. Patients who are given anticoagulant medications should be advised to call whenever they experience a nosebleed. The most common cause of nosebleed is self-induced trauma (picking, rubbing, and nose blowing), often in the context of an allergy, sinusitis, or upper respiratory infection. Dry air, occupational irritants, and nasal recreational drug use predispose to nose bleeding. Systemic disorders that occasionally present as nosebleed include malignant hypertension, bleeding tendencies, and granulomatous diseases. Nosebleed is a rare presentation for malignancy. A key part of the history obtained over the phone is whether the patient is taking medicines, especially anticoagulants such as aspirin or coumadin, or has a chronic bleeding problem such as hemophilia.

Bleeding that occurs in the anterior part of the nostril is usually venous but can be arterial. Bleeding from the posterior part is usually arterial and is more serious. Anterior nosebleed affects one nostril and is often recurrent and moderate in amount. It lasts a short time (10 to 15 minutes) and frequently can be controlled simply by pinching the nostrils. Posterior nosebleed, on the other hand, can affect either one or both nostrils and is brisk. It is difficult to control and requires emergency treatment.

The immediate objective of phone management is to stop the bleeding. Because most nosebleeds are venous and anterior, telling the patient to sit up, lean forward, and compress the nostrils to constrict the flow for 10 to 15 minutes should be effective.

> Bleeding that is brisk, bilateral, or not easily controlled by simple measures such as compression of the nostrils, or bleeding in a patient taking an anticoagulant or one who has a bleeding disorder, is a medical emergency that requires immediate attention.

Before seeing the physician, patients with this more serious posterior bleeding should be instructed to sit up and lean forward but **not** to compress the nostrils, because doing so will cause blood to flow backward into the throat, possibly leading to vomiting and aspiration. These patients need to be seen immediately by a physician skilled in otolaryngologic emergencies for stabilization and usually treatment with topical cocaine, cauterization, or packing.

NOSEBLEED

Question	To See Clinician If . . .	When
1. Patient's name, age, telephone number		
2. Are you taking blood-thinning medicine (Coumadin or long-acting IM heparin)?	Yes, and sitting up, leaning forward, and compression does not stop bleeding in 10 minutes.	2
3. Do you have a history of bleeding problems?	Yes, and sitting up, leaning forward, and compression does not stop bleeding in 10 minutes.	2
4. Is the bleeding from one side of the nose or both sides?	Both sides.	2
	One side.	24-72
5. How much bleeding?		
• More than 1 tsp or full tissue in less than 10 minutes	Brisk bleeding—see if it cannot be stopped.	2
• Less than 1 tsp or full tissue in 10 minutes or more	Moderate bleeding—see only if it recurs.	24-72
6. How long has the bleeding been going on?	More than 1 hour and bleeding is brisk and continuous.	2
	More than 1 hour and bleeding is moderate: see if it recurs.	8
	Less than 1 hour and bleeding is moderate: see if it recurs.	24-72
7. Does the bleeding stop if you sit up, lean forward, and compress the nostrils for 10 minutes?	Yes, but it starts again (moderate bleeding, on one side).	24-72

EMS = Activate EMS SYSTEM		24-72 = Appointment within 3 days	
2 = See ASAP (within 1–2 hours)		72+ = Appointment in 4 days or more	
8 = See same day			

High priority items appear in color.

ADVICE

If the bleeding is moderate and from one side of the nose, the patient should sit up, lean forward, and compress the nostrils for 10 to 15 minutes. If that is ineffective and the patient has no history of bleeding problems and is not taking anticoagulant medication, he or she can try soaking cotton or cloth in Neo-Synephrine or Afrin nose drops if they are available, packing the nostrils with this material, and applying pressure for 5 to 10 minutes. Once the bleeding stops, the patient should apply a lubricant such as petrolatum ointment (for example, Vaseline) or zinc oxide to promote healing. Increasing the level of humidity at home should help to prevent further episodes.

If the bleeding is brisk (especially if it comes from both sides of the nose), or if the patient has a history of bleeding problems or is taking an anticoagulant, the patient should be seen by a skilled physician as soon as possible. In the meantime, these patients should sit up and lean forward, but they should **not** compress the nostrils, because this will cause the blood to flow back into the throat.

A
D
U
L
T

CHAPTER 51

∎∎∎∎∎∎∎∎∎∎∎∎
∎
∎
∎
Rashes and Infestations

Laurence J. Ronan, MD ▪ *Deborah J. Wald, MD*

Adults frequently call to report a new rash. No symptom has a wider differential diagnosis because the same skin manifestations are common to a host of infectious, metabolic, endocrine, and other systemic problems, as well as infestations by insects or mites. The objective of telephone management is to separate out the many self-limited rashes from the few life-threatening rashes or skin warnings of serious systemic illness. Although the odds are great that the rash does not indicate a serious problem, no clinician should feel entirely comfortable until he or she has fully evaluated the rash, including a complete physical examination and appropriate laboratory tests. A few key decision pathways help in determining how quickly this evaluation needs to be done. Telephone attendants also can help patients to control rash symptoms such as itching or pain, attend to cosmetic problems, and prevent spreading and can instruct them on how to get rid of infestations.

Patients have a difficult time describing rashes, but such descriptions are nonetheless worth pursuing. Ask first whether the rash is in one area or widespread. Where is it located (trunk, face, extremities, palms and soles)? Is it progressing through various locations? Generalized petechiae (small, purplish hemorrhagic spots) or other hemorrhagic eruptions may indicate meningococcemia or rickettsial diseases and should prompt immediate attention. So should widespread flat red spots or patches or peeling of the epidermis, which could represent disorders such as toxic shock syndrome. Small, blisterlike elevations (vesicles) suggest the possibility of varicella or herpes zoster. A localized eruption consisting of both raised and flat red spots on the hands or other exposed skin surfaces may indicate a contact dermatitis such as poison ivy or oak or a chemical exposure. Raised, itchy red spots on the lower abdomen (sometimes with bluish-gray spots) may result from the bites of pubic lice (also called crab lice). Small, raised red spots or linear lesions in the armpits, groin, or between the fingers may indicate infestation with a small mite that causes scabies. Eruptions of ulcers or small, firm lumps under the skin (nodules) may indicate a sexually transmitted disease or chronic granulomatous illness.

Patients with a new rash should be asked about fever, muscle or joint pain, and fatigue. The severity and details of a concurrent acute illness suggest how rapidly the clinician needs to see the patient. Patients with symptoms such as intolerance of light or mental status changes (which could indicate meningitis) need emergent attention.

> All rashes in an acutely ill patient who has fever require immediate examination to make a prompt diagnosis in the small number of patients (such as those with septicemia) who need life-saving treatment.

The telephone attendant should elicit a thorough history including past medical problems, current illnesses, medicines, drug allergies, exposures (drugs, travel, sun, sick contacts, pets, wild animals, insect bites, urban versus rural environment, food, and sexual history), and signs of an underlying chronic illness (inflammatory bowel disease, hepatitis, HIV/AIDS, or malignancy). Patients who have immune deficiencies need immediate attention; they may have widespread zoster or sepsis.

Most phone calls, however, are from patients who are not seriously ill but simply are worried about common problems: poison ivy, fungal infections of the groin or foot, contact dermatitis, nonspecific localized eruptions that are itching, or exposure to head lice or another infestation. They are seeking reassurance, relief from pain and itching, quick resolution of a cosmetically disfiguring skin problem, and prevention of further problems. Many can be treated without an office visit. (See the Advice section of this chapter.) Patients with groin rashes should be seen within a few days to rule out more serious problems such as sexually transmitted diseases. Cosmetically important rashes, lesions in the genitalia, and rashes that threaten the eye should not be treated over the phone but should be examined by the clinician, who can make an accurate diagnosis and offer appropriate treatment.

Lice and scabies are not medically dangerous, but they cause patients much anxiety. These common infestations can be difficult to cure if treatment recommendations are not carried out correctly. Patients need calm reassurance and clear instructions over the telephone.

Head lice can occur in patients of any age but are most common in children. Patients may complain of scalp itching or may be asymptomatic. Because most patients have fewer than 10 adult lice, the diagnosis is usually made by identifying the oval-shaped nits, or eggs, which are attached near the base of the hair shaft. Unlike dandruff or flakes of skin, nits are regularly shaped and firmly attached to the hair.

Crab, or pubic, lice are usually found in pubic hair, but now and then are seen in the armpits or eyelashes. This type of louse is slow moving and lives longer than a head louse, so it is more commonly visible. The nits appear as tiny specks on pubic hairs. Patients also get itchy, raised red raised spots at sites of feeding (especially the lower abdomen) and sometimes bluish-gray spots at sites of old bites. Transmission usually requires close physical contact such as sexual intercourse, although sometimes it can occur through contaminated bedding or towels.

Patients with crab lice should come to the office to be evaluated for other sexually transmitted diseases.

Scabies is caused by a small mite that burrows under the skin. Patients develop severe itching once they are sensitized to the mite antigens. Sensitization may take up to 2 or 3 weeks after first exposure, but it happens much more quickly in reinfection. Usually exposure is through close skin-to-skin contact. The mites can survive for more than 2 days on clothing or bedding, however.

The most common symptom of scabies is severe itching. Skin findings usually include small, raised red spots and linear "burrows" in areas such as the armpits, groin, arms, and hands (between the fingers), but skin findings in scabies can be extremely variable. Unless the patient is a known contact of a diagnosed case of scabies, it makes most sense for a patient with suspected scabies to be seen to confirm the diagnosis.

A
D
U
L
T

RASHES

Question	To See Clinician If . . .	When
1. Patient's name, age, telephone number		
2. Do you have any other aches or pains?		
• Neck, eye?	Headache, stiff neck, or avoidance of bright light (meningismus).	EMS
• Joints, chest, etc.?	Joint or muscle pain.	8
3. What does the rash look like?	Generalized petechiae (small, purplish hemorrhagic spots) or other hemorrhagic eruptions.	2
	Generalized itchy, raised red spots (hives, urticaria; see Chapter 31, Allergic Reactions and Anaphylaxis).	2
	Blisters.	8
	Localized eruption consisting of both raised and flat red spots.	24-72
	Raised red spots with linear red "burrows."	24-72
4. Do you have a fever?	Yes, above 101°F.	2
5. Have you been exposed to unusual animals, chemicals, or plants or traveled recently?	Possible tick exposure.	2
	Other plant or animal exposure.	8
6. Where is the rash?	Rash threatens essential organs (eye, mouth, ear).	8
	Rash affects groin or genitals.	24-72
7. Do you have any other medical problems?	Immunocompromised condition: pregnancy, AIDS, cancer, etc.	8
8. Are you taking any new drugs, either prescribed or over the counter?	Yes.	8
9. Have you had close contact with anyone who has been diagnosed with lice or scabies? What type?	Yes—pubic (crab) lice or scabies. (Give home treatment advice for head lice.)	24-72

SEE CHAPTER 31, ALLERGIC REACTIONS AND ANAPHYLAXIS.

EMS	= Activate EMS SYSTEM	24-72	= Appointment within 3 days
2	= See ASAP (within 1–2 hours)	72+	= Appointment in 4 days or more
8	= See same day		

High priority items appear in color.

ADVICE

Rashes

- Moderate contact dermatitis requires removing the offending substance and applying a mild (1%) corticosteroid cream. Occasionally wet dressings with Burow's solution are also helpful.
- Groin rashes may be tinea cruris ("jock itch"), which will respond to over-the-counter antifungal cream, but the patient should see the clinician within a few days to rule out more serious problems such as sexually transmitted diseases.

Head Lice

First, reassure patients that anyone can get head lice—it is not a reflection on their personal hygiene. Then warn them that effective treatment depends on close attention to all three of the following:

- **Shampooing with a louse-killing shampoo.** Several good ones are available without prescription. Permethrin (Nix) has the best activity against both lice and nits. Pyrethrins (RID, A-200) are also effective. Apply to scalp, leave on for 10 minutes, then rinse. Lindane (Quell) requires a prescription and is more toxic. Pregnant or lactating women should not use it. Retreatment may be necessary 7 to 10 days after initial therapy.
- **Removal of nits.** Lice shampoos have always been better at killing adult lice than nits, and there are increasing reports of insect resistance to them. For effective cure, one must physically remove all nits and lice from the hair with a fine-toothed comb. This must be done carefully, methodically, and sometimes repeatedly. Rinsing hair with white vinegar softens and loosens nits, making them easier to remove.
- **Removal from clothing and environment.** Lice can live away from the scalp for up to 55 hours. To prevent reinfection:
  - Machine wash bedding, clothes, and hats. Dry on hot cycle for 20 minutes.
  - Soak combs and brushes in rubbing alcohol or Lysol for 1 hour.
  - Vacuum upholstered furniture, stuffed animals, or other nonwashable items that may have come in close contact with head lice.
  - As an alternative, nonwashable items can be sealed in a plastic garbage bag for 2 weeks.
  - Check and treat all household members and other close contacts.
  - Do not use lice sprays—they are potentially poisonous.

Pubic Lice (Crab Lice)

As for head lice, wash the affected area with permethrin (Nix) 1% cream rinse or pyrethrins/piperonyl butoxide (RID or Innogel), leave on for 10 minutes, then rinse. Lindane is also effective but should not be used by pregnant or lactating women. Nits are generally too tiny to remove. Follow laundry recommendations as above for any contaminated bedding or clothing. Treat all sexual contacts.

Insist that patients with crab lice come to the office to be evaluated for other sexually transmitted diseases. They also should take precautions against spreading the lice until they have been treated.

Scabies

Treatment of scabies requires a prescription, usually permethrin 5% cream (Elimite). Patients should apply the cream all over their skin (from scalp to toes), leave it on for 8 to 14 hours, then wash it off. If they wash their hands during this time, they should reapply the cream to these areas. They should follow the same laundry recommendations as for lice. Close contacts and household members should also be treated if they have symptoms.

It is important to inform patients that persistent itching and rash are common for up to 2 weeks after treatment, owing to a local allergic reaction to dead mites in the skin. This does not mean that the treatment has failed. If symptoms persist beyond 2 weeks, the patient may repeat the same treatment.

CHAPTER 52

■ ■ ■ ■ ■ ■ ■ ■ ■ ■ ■ ■ ■
■
■
⋮

Shortness of Breath (Dyspnea)

John D. Goodson, MD

Shortness of breath (**dyspnea**) is a common experience under conditions of heavy exertion. When it occurs at rest or under unusual circumstances, it is disconcerting at best and alarming at the extreme. Patients reporting shortness of breath may seem excessively anxious, but it is essential to remember that this is a frightening symptom. All patients require a thorough evaluation and the best possible treatment of medical and psychiatric conditions.

> Patients who report shortness of breath require prompt triage because the symptom can point toward impending cardiorespiratory collapse.

Shortness of breath is the sensation that breathing is inadequate to meet body demands. In general, this sensation develops as a result of either inadequate lung or heart function. Lung dysfunction arises when the mechanical activity of the lung is impaired, such as when patients have lost significant lung capacity, or when the actual oxygen/carbon dioxide exchange process in the lung tissue is hindered, such as when the tissue is extensively infected. If heart function is impaired, there may not be sufficient circulation of blood through the lung to meet the body's needs. In addition, if heart function is severely impaired, congestion develops in the blood vessels serving the lungs, which then leads to edema or swelling in the lung tissue itself and decline in lung function. This is a situation known as congestive heart failure. These patients must be identified and treated promptly to prevent respiratory failure.

A marked reduction in blood supply to the heart muscle may cause congestive heart failure and shortness of breath without the chest pain usually associated with angina (see Chapter 35, Chest Pain). These patients also require prompt attention because their shortness of breath may indicate an impending myocardial infarction ("heart attack").

Some medical or psychiatric conditions cause patients to hyperventilate; hyperventilation may be interpreted by the patient as shortness of breath.

The patient who complains of intermittent shortness of breath is reporting the perception that there has been a significant change in activity tolerance. To put this in perspective, it is necessary to ask about the patient's baseline status and the circumstances of symptom development. More frequent symptoms and more dramatic changes will require the fastest attention.

The telephone evaluation of shortness of breath begins with assessment of whether the patient needs emergency treatment.

> If the patient is having difficulty carrying on a phone conversation, prompt attention is mandatory.

If the patient is able to talk comfortably, telephone management should focus on whether the shortness of breath is intermittent, what factors make it better or worse, and whether the patient has any symptoms of infection (e.g., fever or cough), wheezing, or heart disease. It is always useful to ask whether any new or unusual event or exposure occurred before the shortness of breath developed.

Telephone assessment should also include a report of how the patient's level of shortness of breath differs from baseline. Patients with new shortness of breath on minimal activity require evaluation more urgently. Some patients who have chronic shortness of breath will only call when the symptoms become intolerable or are associated with new complaints. Other patients call when shortness of breath develops only in extreme or unusual situations. To put the symptoms in perspective, you should always try to understand the patient's prior experience with shortness of breath, the change from baseline, and the frequency, duration, and severity of symptoms.

Treatment for shortness of breath is based on the identified causes. The chronic diseases that produce shortness of breath are typically those that affect heart or lung function. For patients who have cardiovascular disease, the shortness of breath will resolve when heart function improves. These patients include those with acute coronary artery insufficiency (severe angina), acute myocardial infarction (heart attack), and chronic congestive heart failure. For patients with lung disease, treatment focuses on improving lung function. Mechanical factors include pleural effusions or airway obstruction; lung factors per se include asthma, bronchitis, and pneumonia.

Conditions outside of the heart and lung also can lead to shortness of breath. These range from diabetes (with acidosis) to panic attacks (with hyperventilation).

> In all cases of shortness of breath, the evaluation must initially proceed rapidly, to be sure that the patient does not require emergency care, and thoroughly, to be sure all treatable causes are identified and managed.

Nearly all patients reporting shortness of breath will need to be seen and evaluated by a clinician. The only exception would be for a patient with well-recognized chronic shortness of breath, such as a patient with lung disease who is calling to report a minor change in symptoms.

The decision about when a patient is to be seen should be reviewed with a clinician because additional clinical factors, such as a prior medical condition or previous episodes of shortness of breath, might change the urgency of a follow-up appointment. In some cases, the clinician might ask that the patient be called back to assess any changes in status. If symptoms have accelerated, the urgency of clinical evaluation will increase.

A
D
U
L
T

SHORTNESS OF BREATH (DYSPNEA)

Question	To See Clinician If . . .	When
1. Patient's name, age, telephone number		
2. Are you comfortable with simple conversation?	Uncomfortable (unable to complete sentences).	EMS
	Somewhat uncomfortable (able to complete sentences but feeling short of breath).	2
3. How quickly do you feel that your shortness of breath is worsening?	Rapidly worsening (over the last 12 hours or less).	EMS
	Worsening (over the last 24 hours).	2
	Slowly worsening (over the last 2 to 4 days).	8
4. How long have you been short of breath?	Less than 3 days.	2
	3 to 14 days.	8
	Two weeks or more.	24-72
5. Does your shortness of breath come and go?	No, constant symptoms.	8
	Frequent symptoms (1 to 2 times per week).	8
	Occasional symptoms (1 to 2 times per month).	24-72
6. How much different is your breathing from your usual pattern?	Considerably different (not able to do now what I am usually comfortable doing).	8
	Moderately different (able to do a majority of activities that I am usually comfortable doing).	24-72
	Slightly different (able to do certain activities only with extreme exertion).	72+
7. Are you short of breath only in certain positions, such as when you are on your back?	Yes.	8
8. Do you have a fever over 101.5°F?	Yes.	8

SEE ALSO CHAPTER 61, WHEEZING.

EMS = Activate EMS SYSTEM	**24-72** = Appointment within 3 days
2 = See ASAP (within 1–2 hours)	**72+** = Appointment in 4 days or more
8 = See same day	

High priority items appear in color.

A
D
U
L
T

ADVICE

Most patients with shortness of breath should be seen and evaluated, but the pace of the referral will vary with the situation. Patients with a prior experience of shortness of breath should reinstitute successful treatments as an important first step. Those who also have angina may find that sublingual nitroglycerine will improve symptoms. Those with asthma may be helped by using an inhaler (see Chapter 61, Wheezing).

Patients who have fever with shortness of breath should be told to call back if the fever goes above 101.5°F or if the production of phlegm or sputum increases.

For nearly all patients, slow, steady breathing with an effort to exhale completely with each breath will help to calm the breathing pattern and reduce the risk of hyperventilation. If the patient is having an anxiety attack, establishing rapid contact with a health care provider may be enough to settle the patient and reverse the attack.

CHAPTER 53

Sore Throat

Richard N. Winickoff, MD

Most sore throats in adults are caused by viruses, as they are in children. Likewise, management of sore throat in adults is similar to that in children (see Chapter 25). However, there are some differences. Strep throat is not often recurrent in adults. In fact, it will usually disappear without antibiotics. As in children, the main danger is from the complications of strep throat, such as rheumatic fever and glomerulonephritis, rather than from the strep throat itself. Complications are more likely if the strep is not treated with antibiotics. For this reason, adults with sore throat should be evaluated by the clinician. The clinician may or may not take a throat culture prior to deciding to treat with antibiotics, because clinical features may be as reliable as culture in making a diagnosis in many cases.

In adults there are other diseases that must be considered besides strep and common respiratory viruses.

> Young adults (and occasionally children) may have infectious mononucleosis ("mono"), with or without strep at the same time.

Mono produces severe sore throat and swollen glands, as well as fever, weakness, and depression. It is important to make this diagnosis to inform the patient of the expected duration of mono—much longer than most sore throats—and to make sure the patient avoids contact sports that might result in a ruptured spleen.

Gonorrhea may produce a sore throat that looks very similar to strep. Herpes and yeast also are capable of causing sore throat.

One common type of sore throat is usually associated with a cold virus. If the pain is localized to a small area on one side or the other, and if runny nose and sneezing are present, the problem is usually a cold virus, and there is no need for an office visit. However, if fever or swollen glands are present, the patient should be seen.

In the winter, dry indoor air can be very irritating to the throat. Patients who wake up in the morning with a sore throat that clears after they drink fluids can be advised to obtain a cold- or warm-steam nebulizer for their bedrooms. This approach often improves morning sore throat caused by dryness.

SORE THROAT

Question	To See Doctor If . . .	When
1. Patient's name, age, phone number		
2. Do you have a temperature of more than 100°F?	Yes	8
3. Are your neck glands swollen or tender?	Yes	8
4. Have you had close contact with a person with proven strep throat?	Yes	8
5. Have you had a sore throat continuously for at least 24 hours?	Yes	24-72
6. Are you sneezing or do you have a runny nose?	Yes	24-72

SEE ALSO CHAPTER 36, COLDS AND FLU.

EMS = Activate EMS SYSTEM	24-72 = Appointment within 3 days
2 = See ASAP (within 1–2 hours)	72+ = Appointment in 4 days or more
8 = See same day	

High priority items appear in color.

ADVICE

- If the sore throat is localized to one side and associated with a cold, and there is no fever or swollen glands, the patient may try acetaminophen (Tylenol), 1000 mg every 4 hours for throat pain, along with lozenges, gargles, and hot or cold liquids.
- If the pain occurs only in the morning and it is winter, you could advise the use of a humidifier or steam nebulizer at night. Moistening the air will help the mucous membranes and diminish night and morning distress.

CHAPTER 54

Strains and Sprains

Richard N. Winickoff, MD

Musculoskeletal injuries of the extremities are very common. They can be classified into five categories, in order of increasing seriousness: contusions, strains, sprains, dislocations and fractures.

Contusions

Contusions are the result of blunt trauma that does not involve twisting of joints or breaking of bones. They occur most commonly with falls and blows and are usually seen on exposed surfaces of the arms and legs. They typically start out as swellings with variable amounts of discoloration from bleeding into the tissues. They then become black and blue as the blood is metabolized and the residue is reabsorbed. Contusions are usually tender to touch, but pain is often not increased greatly with function of the extremity unless direct pressure is applied. Contusions resolve fairly rapidly, usually within a week, because the injured structure is not anatomically disrupted in most cases.

Strains

Strains are injuries to muscles and their tendons. Common sites of strains are the shoulder, wrist, and calf. Strains are usually not associated with swelling or discoloration. Tenderness is mild, but pain is elicited when the muscle or tendon is used. Maximum pain is elicited by active motion. A strain occurs when a muscle or tendon is stressed beyond its strength limit and tears. Usually the tear is slight, but it can vary in severity. Muscle strains generally heal quickly, over 1 to 2 weeks, because muscle has a very good blood supply. Tendons heal more slowly, because they are composed of connective tissue with poor blood supply. They usually take 2 to 3 weeks to heal. Tendon strains may develop into tendonitis, a more chronic form of tendon inflammation.

Sprains

Sprains are tears of ligaments that support joints. They are usually caused by twisting injuries. The ankle is the most commonly sprained joint. Wrists, knees, and shoulders may also be sprained. Sprains are often associated with swelling around the joint. Any use of the joint is likely to cause pain, but especially any twisting motion. Weight bearing is moderately painful, but the pain is much more severe with movements that stress the injured ligament. Like tendon strains, sprains often take several weeks to heal.

Dislocations

Dislocations are joints that have been disrupted. They are characterized by displacement of the anatomic relationship of the two bones that make up the joint. A violent injury is usually necessary to cause a dislocation, unless the joint has been previously dislocated. Shoulders are the most commonly dislocated joint, because the cup of the shoulder joint is very shallow to allow full rotation. Fingers are also dislocated frequently.

Fractures

Fractures are broken bones. They occur with severe trauma, such as a fall or a very strong blow to the limb. They are common in football, skiing, or accidents involving bicycles or cars. There may be a deformity of the affected bone. Swelling is usually present, along with bleeding into the tissues. Weight bearing on the affected limb is extremely painful, and indeed the patient may not be able to stand up at all with a lower extremity fracture. Pressure on or around a fracture of the upper extremity is likewise extremely painful.

STRAINS AND SPRAINS

Question	To See Doctor If . . .	When
1. Patient's name, age, telephone number		
2. Are you alert and breathing normally?	No	EMS
3. Are you able to stand?	No	EMS
4. Do you have a lot of pain with weight bearing?	Yes	2
5. Is the injured part swollen or bent in an unusual shape?	Yes	2
6. Is there joint swelling?	Yes	8
7. Is movement of the joint very painful?	Yes	8
8. Is pain only present with certain types of movements?	Yes	24-72
9. Is the only problem swelling and tenderness to touch?	Yes	72+

EMS	= Activate EMS SYSTEM	24-72	= Appointment within 3 days
2	= See ASAP (within 1–2 hours)	72+	= Appointment in 4 days or more
8	= See same day		

High priority items appear in color.

ADVICE

The way that the patient was injured can tell a great deal about the type of injury that is most likely. A direct blow or minor fall is most likely to result in a contusion. If the resultant injury is a swelling without other deformity and does not involve the joint, it is likely to be a contusion. A contusion can be managed safely at home with ice applied for 20 minutes at a time, three or four times daily for 2 or 3 days, and elevation of the affected part as much as possible. Acetaminophen (Tylenol), aspirin, or ibuprofen (Advil, etc.) can be taken to help with pain. If the injury resulted from repeated or excessive use of a particular muscle (such as sawing, swinging a tennis racket, or running very hard), it is likely to be a strain. Activities that irritate the injury should be avoided, and aspirin or ibuprofen should be taken if tolerated, to reduce the inflammation. The physician should be seen only if the injury does not respond to these measures.

If the joint is swollen, the injury is likely to be a sprain, and the patient should be seen. Certain sprains cannot be distinguished from fractures without an x-ray. First aid involves immobilizing the joint with a splint or sling if possible, avoiding weight bearing if the lower extremity is involved and avoiding use if the upper extremity is involved. Ice should be applied to reduce swelling until emergency care can be administered. Patients should go only to facilities that have the capacity to do x-rays.

A patient with inability to bear weight, pain with slight motion of or pressure on the injured area, or deformity of the injured part will need emergency care by an orthopaedic specialist. The primary physician's office should arrange such care directly.

ADULT

CHAPTER 55

■ ■ ■ ■ ■ ■ ■ ■ ■ ■ ■ ■ ■ ■
■
■
Sunburn

Ina Cushman, PA-C

Sunburn is usually a first-degree burn to the skin. The length of sun exposure that causes a burn varies according to personal sensitivity and the intensity of the exposure. The sun's rays are strongest within 2 hours on either side of the brightest sun of the day and are stronger in southern regions, at higher elevations, and near reflective surfaces such as water or snow. Sunburn usually involves injury just to the surface layer of skin, but some tan-promoting agents (especially oils) can produce a more serious burn. Sunburns can occur from the use of tanning booths, which can produce the same detrimental effects as direct sunlight.

Sunburns are characterized by reddened skin that is often warm to the touch due to vasodilatation of the skin vessels. Sometimes blisters can be seen, especially after the use of oils or prolonged sun exposure. Sunburns are often uncomfortable. They are best managed by keeping the area clean with a mild soap and water, using cool compresses on the burned areas, and applying soothing lotions containing aloe vera. Blisters should be left intact.

Simple pain relievers such as acetaminophen or ibuprofen can provide good pain relief if not contraindicated by peptic ulcer disease, allergy, or use of anticoagulants. On rare occasions, patients with more severe pain may need a mild narcotic agent such as codeine for 24 to 48 hours.

Certain medications can make patients more susceptible to sunburn. Some of the common classes of medications with this effect are antibiotics (e.g., trimethoprim/sulfamethoxazole), diuretics (e.g., thiazides, furosemide), and oral antifungal agents (e.g., griseofulvin).

> Patients with sunburn sometimes are also dehydrated, and heat stroke can become a problem. Particularly susceptible are elderly patients and those taking diuretics. Patients who are dehydrated often require intravenous fluids.

The best way to avoid sunburn is to use sunscreens with SPF 15 or greater and to limit unprotected exposure to short periods such as 20 minutes. Sunscreens should be applied 30 minutes before exposure to allow for absorption and they should be reapplied frequently. Clothing with a tight weave will prevent sunburn completely on covered areas of skin.

> SPF is the relative sun protection factor. Theoretically, the higher the number, the longer one can remain in the sun without sunburn. As an example, SPF 15 provides 15 times the natural protection. How many minutes or hours this represents depends on the individual's skin. Sunscreens with an SPF less than 30 protect only from the burning UVB rays of the sun. Sunscreens with SPF of 30 or higher protect from UVA rays as well.

SUNBURN

Question	To See Clinician If . . .	When
1. Patient's name, age, telephone number		
2. Do you have dizziness, confusion, fever, nausea, or decreased urine output?	Yes	2
3. Where is the sunburn? Describe it.	On the face, with swelling or blistering	8
4. Do you have any medical problems?	Diabetes, immune compromise, kidney disease	8
5. Are you taking any medications?	Antibiotics, diuretics (e.g., captopril, hydrochlorothiazide [HCTX], and others), antifungals	8
6. If the sunburn is not a new event, when did it occur? What makes you call now?	Pus coming from blisters	8

EMS = Activate EMS SYSTEM	24-72 = Appointment within 3 days
2 = See ASAP (within 1–2 hours)	72+ = Appointment in 4 days or more
8 = See same day	

High priority items appear in color.

ADVICE

- Cool compresses or cool baths will relieve pain. Patients may use acetaminophen (Tylenol), two 325-mg tablets every 4 to 6 hours or ibuprofen (Advil, etc.), 200 to 400 mg every 4 to 6 hours with food if they have no contraindications.
- Moisturizers (of any kind the patient normally uses) will keep the skin from drying. Some recommend soothing lotions containing aloe vera. These lotions should be kept away from the eyes.
- Patients should drink plenty of fluids to combat dehydration.
- Itching after 2 to 3 days is common. Calamine lotion or an over-the-counter antihistamine (e.g., diphenhydramine [Benadryl] 25 to 50 mg every 6 hours as needed) can be used if the patient has no contraindications.
- Leave blisters intact as long as possible. The top layer will eventually wash off in the shower.
- Watch for pus coming from blisters. The patient should call back if this occurs.

ADULT

CHAPTER 56

Urinary Tract Infections

Jane S. Sillman, MD

Urinary tract infections are common reasons for telephone calls to the physician's office and result in more than seven million office visits annually in the United States. It is important for telephone attendants to know when it is safe to treat a patient over the phone and when to have the patient come in to the office.

Adult patients with urinary tract infections can be classified into five groups:

- Young women with acute uncomplicated bladder inflammation (cystitis)
- Young women with recurrent cystitis
- Young women with acute uncomplicated inflammation of the kidney and ureter (pyelonephritis)
- All adults with complicated urinary tract infections
- Adults with bacteria in the urine, without symptoms

Adults in the first four groups are apt to call with symptoms of pain or burning on urination (dysuria). Ideally, all of these patients should be seen in the office. Young women with acute uncomplicated cystitis who are unable to come in often can be safely treated over the phone, however, so it is the task of the telephone attendant to determine which group a patient belongs in and what the next step in evaluation should be.

Young women calling with the recent onset of burning on urination often have acute uncomplicated cystitis, but it is possible that they could have an acute inflammation of the urethra (urethritis) due to chlamydia, gonorrhea, or herpes, or they could have inflammation of the vagina due to candida or trichomonas. The presenting symptoms can be helpful in making the correct diagnosis. With acute cystitis, the painful urination usually comes on quickly and the patient also may have urinary frequency and urgency and blood in the urine. With acute urethritis, the symptoms more often come on gradually and are milder; these patients often have a vaginal discharge or vaginal bleeding as well. They may report having a new sexual partner. Patients with vaginitis often report external burning on urination, vaginal discharge or odor, vaginal itch, painful intercourse, and no increased urinary frequency or urgency.

About 80% of cases of cystitis are due to E. coli, with a few other organisms causing most of the remaining cases. These organisms are usually sensitive to trimethoprim-sulfamethoxazole and fluoroquinolones. Because of this predictability, a urine culture is generally not needed and a 3-day course of antibiotic treatment can be recommended. A pretreatment culture and a 7-day course of treatment are recommended instead, however, for patients with certain risk factors:

- Pregnancy
- Diabetes
- Symptoms for more than 7 days

- Use of a diaphragm
- Age greater than 65 years

If a patient's history is classic for cystitis, she does not have a vaginal discharge or a new sexual partner, she has none of the risk factors just listed, and she is unable to come to the office, it is reasonable to ask the clinician about prescribing a 3-day course of antibiotics over the phone. The patient should be told to call back to arrange for an appointment if her symptoms do not completely resolve after 3 days of treatment. In general, however, it is preferable to see all women with cystitis in the office to confirm the diagnosis.

About 20% of young women have recurrent cystitis, with episodes occurring months apart, owing to reinfection rather than persistence of infection. Risk factors for recurrent infections include sexual intercourse and use of a diaphragm and spermicide. Recurrent infection should be confirmed by culture at least once.

In postmenopausal women, recurrent episodes of cystitis may be the result when the bladder or uterus falls out of position, causing urine to be left in the bladder after urination. Another cause may be thinning and inflammation of vaginal tissues associated with increased populations of E. coli. These patients need to be seen for a pelvic exam and urine culture.

Young women with acute uncomplicated pyelonephritis (kidney inflammation) typically report symptoms of fever and flank pain in addition to dysuria. All such patients should be seen promptly. Many can be treated with antibiotics as outpatients, but some require hospitalization.

Complicated urinary tract infections are defined as those occurring in a patient who has an abnormal urinary tract or those due to antibiotic-resistant organisms. These patients (both men and women) may be mildly to severely ill and may be infected with a wide range of organisms. All patients suspected of having a complicated urinary tract infection need an office assessment. All urinary tract infections in men aged 50 or older are considered to be complicated infections.

Men younger than 50 may develop uncomplicated cystitis due to E. coli. In addition to dysuria, symptoms may include discharge from the urethra, so the evaluation must include testing for gonorrhea, chlamydia, and herpes as well as a urine culture. Risk factors for cystitis in young men include anal intercourse and being uncircumcised.

Patients with urinary catheters should be treated for symptomatic episodes of infection based on the results of urine cultures. If they have no symptoms, treatment is not recommended.

A
D
U
L
T

URINARY TRACT INFECTIONS

Question	To See Clinician If . . .	When
1. Patient's name, age, telephone number		
2. What are your symptoms? Burning or pain on urination? Frequency or urgency of urination?	If patient answers No to questions 4–9 and has had symptoms for less than 7 days, prescribing treatment over the phone is possible, though a same-day visit to the office (or lab, for urinalysis) is preferable.	
3. How long have the symptoms been present?	7 days or more.	8
4. Do you have a fever?	Yes.	8
5. Do you have back pain?	Yes.	8
6. Have you had a urinary tract infection in the past year?	Yes.	8
7. (If the patient is female) Do you have a vaginal discharge?	Yes.	8
8. Do you have a new sexual partner?	Yes.	8
9. Are you nauseated or vomiting?	Yes.	8
10. Do you have any drug allergies?		

EMS	= Activate EMS SYSTEM	24-72	= Appointment within 3 days
2	= See ASAP (within 1–2 hours)	72+	= Appointment in 4 days or more
8	= See same day		

High priority items appear in color.

ADVICE

Young women with symptoms consistent with acute uncomplicated cystitis and no other risk factors may be treated with an antibiotic prescribed without an office visit (although a visit is preferable). These patients should be told to call the office and request a same-day appointment if their symptoms have not resolved by the third day of treatment.

It is helpful to give advice about preventing future episodes of cystitis. Patients whose symptoms appear to be related to recent sexual activity should void after intercourse. Those who are using a diaphragm with spermicide have an increased risk of urinary tract infections and may want to consider switching to another method of contraception.

CHAPTER 57

■■■■■■■■■■■■
■
■
Vaginal Bleeding

Martin A. Quan, MD

Abnormal vaginal bleeding, defined as any vaginal bleeding that is not consistent with normal menstruation, is a common gynecologic problem that is likely to occur in most women at some point during their reproductive lives. Normal menstruation occurs at intervals of 21 to 39 days and lasts from 2 to 7 days, with a volume of blood loss ranging from 29 to 60 mL (1 to 2 ounces). Telephone management of this condition is driven primarily by three factors: (1) the impact of the bleeding on the patient's cardiovascular system, (2) the rate of vaginal bleeding currently present, and (3) the diagnostic and therapeutic implications raised by the underlying condition.

Abnormal vaginal bleeding can have many causes, some of which are listed on Table 57–1. Bleeding that is not related to a complication of pregnancy is seldom life threatening. Nevertheless, you should ask about signs suggesting low blood pressure and cardiovascular instability, because their presence would indicate an emergency.

> Symptoms of fainting, lightheadedness, or dizziness when upright all suggest a significant amount of blood loss and call for immediate evaluation and management.

TABLE 57-1 Causes of Abnormal Vaginal Bleeding
Dysfunctional uterine bleeding (without ovulation)
Pregnancy-related causes (e.g., ectopic pregnancy, spontaneous abortion, gestational trophoblastic disease)
Anatomic gynecologic disorders
Vulvovaginal (neoplasms, trauma, foreign bodies)
Cervical (polyps, cancer, cervicitis)
Endometrial (pelvic inflammatory disease, uterine fibroids, adenomyosis, atrophic endometrium, polyps, hyperplasia, cancer)
Ovarian (neoplasms)
Iatrogenic
Hormonal contraception
Intrauterine contraceptive device
Anticoagulant therapy
Hormone replacement therapy
Recent surgery
Systemic
Endocrine disorders (thyroid disorders, diabetes, adrenal disorders)
Chronic liver disease
Chronic renal disease
Coagulation disorders

If the patient has none of those symptoms, the rate of bleeding should then be gauged.

> If the patient reports the passage of watery, bright red blood, especially if it requires the use of one pad or more per hour to absorb, quick evaluation for severe bleeding is needed.

The passage of blood clots also suggests heavy bleeding and requires urgent evaluation.

Apart from considerations related directly to the severity of bleeding, the likely cause of the bleeding also affects telephone management of the patient. The consequences of certain disorders that produce vaginal bleeding can be worsened by delays in therapy. Among these are disorders related to infections, including pelvic inflammatory disease, endometritis, and infectious cervicitis. They usually can be identified because they are accompanied by pain.

Pregnancy-related conditions are the most common causes of life-threatening vaginal bleeding. Patients with vaginal bleeding should thus be routinely asked whether they are known to be pregnant and, if the answer is no, about the likelihood that they may be pregnant. This can be assessed by inquiring about their last menstrual period, their level of sexual activity, and, if sexually active, their method of contraception. Vaginal bleeding related to a complication of pregnancy (e.g., ectopic pregnancy, spontaneous abortion, any bleeding occurring in the second half of pregnancy) requires immediate attention regardless of its severity.

VAGINAL BLEEDING

Question	To See Clinician If . . .	When
1. Patient's name, age, telephone number		
2. When did your bleeding begin? When was your last menstrual period?	If patient who had been menstruating is late for her period, see question 7.	
3. Do you feel faint, lightheaded, or unsteady when you stand?	Yes.	EMS
4. Are you passing watery, bright red blood requiring more than one pad an hour?	Yes.	EMS
5. Are you passing clots?	Yes.	2
6. Is the bleeding associated with pain?	Yes.	8
7. Are you pregnant? If not certain, are you sexually active and not using a reliable method of birth control?	Yes. If not certain, obtain pregnancy test and see same day if positive.	8
8. Is the bleeding in excess of your normal menstrual flow?	Yes.	24-72
9. Have you experienced menopause?	Yes.	72+
10. Has the bleeding stopped or are you just experiencing spotting?	Yes.	72+

SEE ALSO CHAPTER 48, MENSTRUAL PAIN.

EMS = Activate EMS SYSTEM	24-72	= Appointment within 3 days
2 = See ASAP (within 1–2 hours)	72+	= Appointment in 4 days or more
8 = See same day		

High priority items appear in color.

A
D
U
L
T

ADVICE

Until medical assistance arrives, the patient who feels light-headed or faint should

- Lie down on her back
- Elevate her feet higher than her head
- Loosen belt, collar, or other constrictive clothing

Make sure that the patient understands that pregnancy-related causes of vaginal bleeding require urgent attention, so it is important to find out whether she is pregnant. The results of a properly performed home pregnancy test are helpful, especially if she is more than 1 week late for her period.

It is also useful to assess the amount of bleeding, so the patient should keep track of how many pads or tampons are used (although such assessments are often unreliable). Abnormally heavy menstrual bleeding is usually defined as bleeding that requires more than 10 to 15 pads or tampons per period. Whether the toilet water looks pink is not a good indicator of severity because even a drop of blood will make the water pink.

CHAPTER 58

Vaginal Discharge

Phyllis L. Carr, MD

Vaginal discharge is a common medical problem in women, resulting in 5 to 10 million office visits a year in the United States. It commonly stems from one of three infectious causes:

- Yeast
- An overgrowth of certain bacteria (bacterial vaginosis)
- Trichomonas (a protozoan)

All three can cause significant discomfort as well as complications in certain situations. Accurate diagnosis and treatment are essential for effective management.

Normal, physiologic secretions of the vagina include cervical mucous and other substances secreted by several glands. These secretions ordinarily pool in the posterior fornix of the vagina and do not adhere to the vaginal walls. An abnormal discharge is usually accompanied by irritation, itching, odor, or urinary symptoms such as burning or frequency. The discharge can range from thick to watery and frothy, and from white to yellow, gray, or green.

> When a woman has a vaginal infection, the objectives of management are twofold: to make the patient comfortable and to obtain an accurate diagnosis so that appropriate treatment can be initiated.

Yeast

A yeast infection affects most adult women at least once during their lifetime. Severe itching or irritation can affect both the vagina and the vulvar area, as well as the skin folds of the groin. The appearance of the odorless discharge ranges from thick and white to a yellow "cottage cheese" appearance. Over-the-counter treatments are appropriate if the woman has had exactly the same symptoms diagnosed as a yeast infection in the past—but not too recently; if the interval has been less than a month, the same infection may be recurring. Suppositories are effective when the symptoms affect mostly the vaginal area; if they are more widespread, a cream is better. Prescription therapy should be used for a recurrence or if the patient has already been treated with an over-the-counter treatment that was ineffective.

Bacterial Vaginosis

An overgrowth of certain bacterial species, along with a decrease in normal vaginal flora, is a frequent cause of vaginal inflammation. The discharge is thin and a homogeneous gray to white color, with a prominent fishy odor. Half of patients have no symptoms, and the vulvar area and groin are not involved. This condition can be associated with complications such as an abnormal Pap smear, infections of the upper genital tract, and premature rupture of membranes and premature delivery in pregnancy.

Treatment involves prescribing an antibiotic given two to three times a day for 7 days, either orally or topically. There is a one-dose treatment, but it has been associated with a higher rate of recurrence, so the longer course is preferred for patients who are likely to comply with it.

Trichomonas

The incidence of trichomonas infections has been declining, but it still accounts for between 10 and 25% of vaginal infections. The infection is transmitted sexually, and the rate is higher among patients seen in sexually transmitted disease clinics. It is more likely in patients who have a greater number of sexual partners, those who smoke cigarettes, and African Americans, even after adjustment for income and level of education. Sometimes patients have both trichomonas infection and bacterial vaginosis.

Between 25 and 50% of women with trichomonas infections have no symptoms. Some have itching, but the vulva and groin are not affected. The discharge is generally profuse, watery, frothy, and green, with a bad odor. As with bacterial vaginosis, complications can include an abnormal Pap smear, infections of the upper genital tract, and premature rupture of membranes and premature delivery in pregnancy.

Trichomonas infection is treated with a prescription antibiotic given orally either in a one-time dose or two to three times a day for 7 days. The sexual partner should be treated as well. In pregnancy, the one-time dose is used and the patient is followed up to be certain of cure.

VAGINAL DISCHARGE

Question	To See Clinician If . . .	When
1. Patient's name, age, telephone number		
2. Do you have burning or frequency of urination?	Yes.	8
3. Do you have a fever, nausea, or abdominal pain?	Yes.	8
4. Is there blood in the discharge (if not having menstrual period)?	Yes.	8
5. What is the discharge like? Does it have an odor? Is there itching and discomfort?	Discharge is thick and white with little or no odor. Patient is very uncomfortable.	8
	Discharge is thick and white with little or no odor. Minimal discomfort.	24-72
	Discharge is thin, with bad odor.	24-72
6. How long have you had the symptoms? Have you used over-the-counter medications for them?	More than a week and/or have used OTC medications.	24-72
7. Is there any chance that you could be pregnant?	Yes (no symptoms from questions 2–4).	24-72
8. Have you had a new sexual partner recently, or could you have been exposed to a sexually transmitted disease?	Yes.	24-72
9. Have you had very similar symptoms before, more than a month ago?	Yes—OTC medication can be tried.	

EMS = Activate EMS SYSTEM
2 = See ASAP (within 1–2 hours)
8 = See same day
24-72 = Appointment within 3 days
72+ = Appointment in 4 days or more

High priority items appear in color.

ADULT

ADVICE

- Treatment of vaginal discharge over the telephone is only appropriate for patients who have previously been evaluated in the office for yeast infections, who had a rapid response to treatment, and who have exactly the same symptoms. Patients who are taking prednisone (steroids) or oral contraceptives or who have recently completed a course of antibiotics are likely to fall into this category.
- Over-the-counter treatments for these patients include miconazole (Monistat) 100-mg vaginal suppositories or 2% vaginal cream nightly for 7 to 10 days, or clotrimazole (Gyne-Lotrimin) 100-mg vaginal suppositories or 1% vaginal cream nightly for 7 to 10 days. Shorter-course treatments such as clotrimazole 100-mg vaginal suppositories twice a day for 3 days are also available but have a higher relapse rate. The suppositories are effective for symptoms limited to the vaginal area, but the creams are better if itching is widespread. All patients using these medications should be instructed to call back for an appointment if the symptoms do not go away within 3 to 5 days after starting treatment.
- Patients who need an office visit should stop using any vaginal medications at least 24 hours before their appointment.

CHAPTER 59

∎ ∎ ∎ ∎ ∎ ∎ ∎ ∎ ∎ ∎ ∎ ∎

Visual Disturbance

Richard S. Weinhaus, MD

Two common conditions causing a visual disturbance may lead patients to phone in. One is visual migraine and the other is shifting of the vitreous gel inside the eye, which causes flashes of light, "floaters," or both. Although patients may use terms like "flashes of light" or "flashing lights" to describe both conditions, almost all patients can be properly triaged on the basis of the phone history alone.

Visual Migraine

The hallmark of a visual migraine is a **continuous** visual disturbance that usually lasts about 10 to 30 minutes and then resolves. The visual disturbance is described as being active—for example, shimmering, jagged, like a kaleidoscope, or like neon lights. In some cases, the center of the jagged or shimmering disturbance becomes a blind spot, which may slowly migrate across the visual field. Patients who were reading or driving may report that they had to stop because they could not see.

> The visual disturbance usually involves either the left or the right side of visual space in **both** eyes (that is, the left or the right visual field), but patients may incorrectly perceive the former as being in the left eye and the latter as being in the right eye. If the patient is asked to close each eye in turn, he or she may be able to confirm that the disturbance is in both eyes.

As the visual phenomena begin to recede, they often are followed by a severe throbbing headache, nausea, and sensitivity to bright lights and loud noises. If these symptoms are present, it clinches the diagnosis of migraine. It is not uncommon, however, for a patient to have the visual portion of a migraine without the other symptoms or with just a mild headache. This is called a migraine equivalent. If the patient has had previous identical episodes, even months or years before, this helps confirm the diagnosis of migraine.

Visual migraines are benign and the patient may be reassured by phone. They can be frightening, however, especially if the patient has not experienced one before.

Nonmigrainous Causes of Sudden Visual Loss

A sudden decrease in central or peripheral vision that has not cleared within an hour suggests a serious problem of the optic nerve, retina, or central nervous system and needs to be evaluated urgently.

Amaurosis fugax is a **temporary** visual disturbance in one eye. It is a rare condition and is usually caused by a partially blocked carotid artery (the major artery in the neck that supplies the eye and brain). This condition almost always occurs only in older patients who have risk factors for cerebrovascular disease. The classic description is that of a "shade" coming down over one eye so that everything blacks out. After about 5 minutes, the shade gradually lifts. There are no shimmering, jagged, or colorful lights as are described with visual migraine and no flashes or floaters. Amaurosis fugax is a form of transient ischemic attack (TIA) and should be evaluated with the same urgency as other TIAs.

Flashes and Floaters

The retina is the flat sheet of tissue covering the inner back wall of the eye. It does the actual seeing, like the film in a camera. The vitreous gel is the nearly transparent, jelly-like substance that fills most of the volume of the eye. In the young eye, the vitreous gel is firmly attached to the retina. However, with age, nearsightedness (myopia), recent head or eye trauma, or cataract surgery, the gel may begin to pull away from the retina in certain areas. When the eye or head moves, this loose gel tugs on the adjacent attached gel, which in turn tugs on the retina. But the retina does not have any way of sensing these tugs as tugs. Rather, it perceives them as flashes of light. There is no pain or pulling sensation.

In contrast to the **continuous** "flashing lights" reported in migraine, tugging on the retina by the vitreous gel causes brief, **intermittent,** lightning-like flashes. The flashes may be frequent, but each one only lasts for a second. The flashes are often described as being arcs or semicircles of light, off to the side. These retinal flashes are induced by turning the eye or the head and appear in only one eye. Patients are more aware of retinal flashes in the dark, because there are fewer competing visual stimuli.

After a period of hours to days, the back surface of the vitreous gel usually completely pulls away from the retina (a vitreous detachment). The perception of flashes ceases and is replaced by what the patient describes as a floating hair or specks, a cobweb, a transparent cloud, or a fly or bug. Some patients may tell you that at first they reached out with their hand to try to grab the floating object. They always fail, of course, because what they are really seeing is the back portion of the vitreous gel floating around inside the eye. Many patients experience vitreous floaters without having had any preceding flashes of light.

The new onset of flashes or floaters due to a vitreous detachment is annoying and anxiety provoking, but is not usually a serious problem. In a few cases, however, the vitreous gel is so firmly attached to the retina that when it pulls away, it causes a retinal tear; an actual flap of torn retina remains attached to the floating vitreous gel. Because the gel continues to tug on the torn flap of retina, the patient usually continues to have flashes in addition to floaters.

Unless a retinal tear is sealed by a laser or freezing treatment, the liquid portion of the vitreous gel may seep underneath the retina, causing the retina itself to balloon forward or detach. This is called a **retinal detachment.** Patients will be aware of a visual field defect, which they may describe as a shadow blocking a portion of their vision.

Retinal tears and retinal detachments are urgent conditions. If a patient calls complaining of the new onset of flashes or floaters, you can assume that they have developed a vitreous detachment, but you cannot sort out by history whether a retinal tear is present. Anything in the vitreous gel, including hemorrhage, inflammatory cells, or benign clumps of the gel itself, will also cause floaters. All patients with flashes or floaters need to be seen by an eye specialist, who will perform a dilated retinal exam. If flashes persist, patients should be seen urgently, and if they report a visual field defect, they need to be seen very urgently by a specialist. A visit to a primary care practitioner or the emergency room is a wasted visit.

VISUAL DISTURBANCE

Question	To See Clinician If . . .	When
1. Patient's name, age, telephone number		
2. Has the problem with your vision lasted for more than 1 hour?	If Yes, go to question 3. If No, go to question 7.	
3. Is there anything that looks like a fly or hair floating around inside your eye? If so, how long has it been present?	Yes (all should be seen by an eye specialist): • Present less than 1 week. • Present several weeks. • Unchanged for months or years.	8 24-72 72+
4. Do you see a brief flash of light off to the side when you turn your eye or your head? If so, how long has it been present?	Yes (all patients with normal vision and brief, intermittent flashes in one eye should be seen by an eye specialist): • Present less than 1 week. • Present several weeks. • Unchanged for months or years.	8 24-72 72+
5. Have you lost a portion of your peripheral or central vision in one eye?	Yes (rare; suggests retinal detachment or other serious problem).	2
6. Do you have • Severe nearsightedness? • A history of retinal tear or detachment? • A history of recent eye or head trauma? • A history of cataract surgery or other eye surgery?	Yes to any (risk factors for retinal tear or detachment).	8

Visual Migraine

Question	To See Clinician If . . .	When
7. Did it seem as if a shade came down over just one eye, causing the vision to go totally dark for about 5 minutes?	Yes (suggestive of a TIA).	8
8. Did you see jagged, shimmering, or kaleidoscopic images?	No. (If Yes, probably migraine; reassure patient.)	24-72
9. Do you have a history of heart attack, stroke, or other serious medical problem?	Yes (urgency depends on history and symptoms).	

EMS = Activate EMS SYSTEM

2 = See ASAP (within 1–2 hours)

8 = See same day

24-72 = Appointment within 3 days

72+ = Appointment in 4 days or more

High priority items appear in color.

ADVICE

Many patients with their first episode of visual migraine are concerned that they may be developing a retinal detachment or a stroke, especially if they have no other migrainous symptoms. If the visual disturbance has resolved within an hour and is consistent with a migraine, reassure the patient. If migrainous episodes are very frequent, encourage the patient to make an appointment with the primary care clinician.

Patients with new onset of floaters or flashes suggesting vitreous detachment need to be seen urgently by an eye specialist. These patients should call before the time of their appointment if they develop an increase in flashes, a new shower of floaters, or a shadow in a portion of their vision.

Patients who have episodes of vague or ambiguous visual disturbances should keep a log documenting how often the episodes occur, how long they last, and whether there are any other associated symptoms. They should cover each eye in turn to determine whether the visual problem is in just one eye or in both eyes. This information will be of great help in sorting out the problem.

CHAPTER 60

Vomiting and Nausea

David E. Katz, MD ▪ *William F. Kelly III, MD*
Christopher P. Cheney, MD, PhD

Vomiting is the forceful expulsion of stomach contents. **Nausea** is the unpleasant sensation that vomiting is about to occur. Vomiting should be distinguished from **retching,** muscle contractions without vomiting (also called dry heaves), and **regurgitation,** the reflux of ingested material into the patient's mouth without nausea or contractions. Vomiting is a complex process involving two areas of the brain, the chemoreceptor trigger zone and the vomiting center. These centers coordinate chest and abdominal muscle contractions during the process of vomiting.

> Vomiting complications include dehydration, metabolic disturbances, injury to the esophagus, malnutrition, aspiration, and dental problems.

Treatment includes preventing or correcting dehydration, making dietary changes, and often administering medication.

Causes

Drugs are the most common cause of nausea and vomiting in elderly patients (e.g., aspirin and other analgesics, alcohol, digitalis, iron, steroids, antibiotics, or chemotherapy). They cause intestinal irritation and also may stimulate the vomiting centers in the brain.

Neurological causes include alterations in the vestibular system (balance problems and motion sickness), brain tumors, strokes, meningitis, and migraine headaches.

Infections caused by viruses or bacterial toxins associated with food poisoning are a common cause of nausea and vomiting.

Most **pregnant** women have nausea in the first trimester, and about half experience vomiting. Hyperemesis gravidarum is a term used when symptoms are severe.

Gastrointestinal disorders that can be associated with vomiting include peptic ulcer disease (most often associated with helicobacter pylori infection), appendicitis, pancreatitis, perforation, kidney stones, small bowel obstruction (from cancer, surgical scars, or hernias), or stool impaction. Some of these may require surgical intervention.

Vomiting also can be a symptom of **electrolyte abnormalities,** as seen in kidney failure. **Psychiatric disorders, heart attacks,** and **glaucoma** may be associated with nausea and vomiting, as can long-standing **diabetes** (e.g., more than 20 years), from loss of normal gastric emptying.

> Most cases of vomiting resolve spontaneously. In over half of the cases, no clear cause can be found.

VOMITING AND NAUSEA

Question	To See Clinician If . . .	When
1. Patient's name, age, telephone number		
2. How many times have you vomited over the last 24 hours?		
3. What did the vomit contents look like?	Blood, black, or "coffee grounds."	EMS
4. Did you hit your head prior to vomiting? Did you lose consciousness?	Yes to either.	EMS
5. Do you have abdominal pain or fever?	Pain is severe (bending over with discomfort) or temperature is greater than 101°F.	2
6. Do you have a headache?	Stiff neck, eyes sensitive to light, fever, worst headache of patient's life.	2
7. Do you have any signs of dehydration? • Lightheaded when standing? • Dark yellow urine or no urine output for 8 to 10 hours? • Skin remains "tented" when lightly pinched? (Pinch a fold of loose skin on the abdomen and release. Is the skin delayed in returning to its normal position?) • Unable to keep any liquids down for more than 24 hours? • Having trouble thinking or concentrating?	Yes.	8
8. Is your head spinning or are you losing your balance?	Yes.	8
9. Are you being treated for cancer with medications?	Yes.	8
10. Are you having multiple loose stools (more than 3 per day)?	Yes.	8
11. Have you been binge drinking?	Yes.	8
12. Have you been told that you have gallstones?	Yes.	8
13. Is your skin yellow?	Yes.	8
14. Is anyone else at your home vomiting?	Yes.	24-72
15. Do you have any other serious or chronic medical conditions?	Diabetes, kidney stones, cancer, current infection, history of hernia or abdominal surgery, no bowel movements.	24-72
16. Are you taking medications?	Narcotics, aspirin/analgesics, digitalis, iron, steroids, antibiotics, chemotherapy.	8

VOMITING AND NAUSEA (Continued)

Question	To See Clinician If . . .	When
17. Were you exposed to food that may have been spoiled? (e.g., picnic food: potato salad or mayonnaise products)	Yes.	24-72
18. Are you or could you be pregnant (any menstrual period irregularities)?	Yes.	72+

EMS = Activate EMS SYSTEM	24-72	= Appointment within 3 days
2 = See ASAP (within 1–2 hours)	72+	= Appointment in 4 days or more
8 = See same day		

High priority items appear in color.

ADVICE

The most important principle is to identify the occasional serious condition. After this, the best home management is to avoid dehydration by drinking as much fluid as possible without making symptoms worse. If an office visit is not indicated, advise the patient to:

• Watch urine color and output. Dark urine and minimal output may be associated with dehydration.
• Drink until urinating every few hours or until urine is clear or very light yellow.
• Start with water, ginger ale, or ice chips. If tolerated, advance to thicker liquids like broths, soups, and gelatins. Then try solid foods such as crackers and, finally, a normal diet.
• Avoid sugar-free (diet) products and milk products.
• Not start or stop medicines without consulting the doctor.

   Medication to stop vomiting is occasionally needed. Common medications include:

• **Diphenhydrinate (Dramamine):** available over the counter, 50 mg every 4 hours, by mouth as needed.
• **Prochlorperazine (Compazine):** available by prescription, 5 to 10 mg every 6 to 8 hours by mouth or IM shot as needed. Available as a 25-mg suppository given every 12 hours as needed.
• **Promethazine (Phenergen):** available by prescription, 25 to 50 mg every 4 to 6 hours by mouth or IM shot as needed. Available as a 12.5-, 25-, or 50-mg suppository given every 12 hours as needed.

   Common adverse reactions to these medications include drowsiness, dizziness, blurred vision, skin rash, hypotension, and neuromuscular reactions. Alternative remedies, including herbs and acupuncture, are sometimes used.

   Remind patients that they should always consult a doctor before starting or stopping any medication.

   Always advise the patient to call back if symptoms continue or worsen.

A
D
U
L
T

CHAPTER 61

Wheezing

John D. Goodson, MD

Wheezing describes a breathing pattern that arises when the flow in the airways is obstructed. It is accompanied by a high-pitched sound that coincides with inspiration, expiration, or both. Wheezing is a hallmark of asthma (a condition in which various stimuli cause constriction of the bronchial airways), although some patients with severe asthma cannot move enough air to cause audible wheezing. For some, wheezing is a chronic condition that becomes an accepted part of life, whereas for others it is a new experience that may be frightening and cause considerable apprehension. Experienced patients may refer to their wheezing as "my asthma."

Telephone management should focus on the following: the acuteness of the patient's symptoms; the patient's prior experience and treatment of wheezing or asthma; the patient's other medical conditions; exposure to toxins, medications, allergens, or irritants; the presence of infection; and the patient's level of apprehension. Any condition that interferes with normal respiration can be potentially dangerous and can create a sense of desperation in the patient.

> The telephone interaction can help to calm the patient, even one who is wheezing severely, by reassuring him or her that treatment is available and effective.

Wheezing generally develops as a consequence of airway obstruction. With some patients, the symptoms are intermittent, pointing toward a process that waxes and wanes; for others, symptoms are persistent. In either group, symptoms can be progressive over short time periods. The airway can be obstructed at any level and the obstruction can be focal or diffuse. Focal obstruction occurs in or adjacent to a large airway. Diffuse obstruction can occur at any level, although symptomatic obstruction most commonly develops in the small airways of the lung.

Focal airway obstruction may be a consequence of mechanical factors, such as aspirated food; infections, such as epiglottitis; or tumor, such as bronchogenic cancer.

Diffuse obstruction can develop in the small airways as a consequence of allergy, infection, irritation, exposure to a toxic substance, inflammation, vascular congestion, or chronic lung disease. Some individuals have a very high level of airway reactivity and are very prone to airway obstruction and wheezing. Because some conditions can lead to a rapid decline of lung function, patients with rapidly deteriorating lung function require immediate attention.

> Telephone assessment should identify the situation in which the symptoms developed, any associated precipitants, the pace and frequency of wheezing, and the patient's comfort level.

   Treatment for wheezing depends on the location of the obstruction. If the obstruction is focal, treatment or removal of the obstruction produces relief. If the process is diffuse, treatment must stabilize the obstruction and ensure sufficient lung function for patient comfort. In some cases, this merely involves removing a toxic or noxious agent. In others it involves systemic therapy to treat a diffuse inflammatory process in the lungs. In all cases, the pace of treatment is contingent on the virulence of the process and the patient's pulmonary reserve. For patients with some conditions, such as hyperactive airways or severe infection, rapid and aggressive therapy is needed to prevent respiratory collapse. In patients who have limited lung capacity to begin with, even relatively minor obstruction can cause a dangerous decline in lung function. The primary clinician should be involved in determining the timing of the evaluation of such patients.

   The patient's prior experience with wheezing can help to guide telephone management. Some patients can specifically outline the treatment protocol that has served them best in the past. In these situations, the patient's experience and request should be recorded and reviewed with the clinician.

   Patients who breathe comfortably in normal daily activities but have intermittent wheezing may require extensive evaluation to determine a specific cause. Some of these patients can be followed expectantly with instructions to call and to be seen when symptoms are present.

WHEEZING

Question	To See Clinician If . . .	When
1. Patient's name, age, telephone number		
2. How severe is your wheezing?	Very severe (constant difficulty with all activities)	`EMS`
	Severe (difficulties with most activities)	`8`
	Moderate (difficulties with some daily activities)	`24-72`
	Mild (intermittent symptoms or mild symptoms and no limitation of daily activities)	`72+`
3. How quickly do you feel that your wheezing is worsening?	Severely (worse over last 24 hours)	`2`
	Moderately (worse over last 24 to 72 hours)	`8`
	Mildly (worse over last several days)	`24-72`
4. How long has this episode of wheezing been going on?	Less than 2 weeks	`8`
	More than 2 weeks	`24-72`
5. Before this episode, have you had trouble with your lungs?	Very severe (constant difficulty with most activities)	`2`
	Severe (difficulties with most activities)	`8`
	Moderate (difficulties with some daily activities)	`24-72`
	Mild (intermittent or mild symptoms and no difficulties with daily activities)	`72+`
6. Do you have fever? Cough (with or without phlegm)?	Yes	`8`
7. Does your wheezing come and go?	No, constant symptoms	`8`
	Frequent episodes (1 to 2 per week)	`24-72`
	Occasional episodes (1 to 2 per month)	`72+`

SEE ALSO CHAPTER 35, CHESTPAIN.

`EMS`	= Activate EMS SYSTEM	`24-72`	= Appointment within 3 days
`2`	= See ASAP (within 1–2 hours)	`72+`	= Appointment in 4 days or more
`8`	= See same day		

High priority items appear in color.

A
D
U
L
T

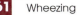

ADVICE

If the patient is wheezing heavily during the telephone conversation, ask the patient to be sure to blow each breath out as much as possible before drawing the next breath. This should pace the respirations slightly. It also may be helpful for the patient to purse the lips slightly (as if blowing out a candle) while exhaling each breath. These measures can help to settle the patient somewhat, although most with this level of wheezing will need care as quickly as it can be arranged. If the wheezing is accelerating, impress on the patient that care must be obtained immediately. Notify the clinician (interrupting if necessary) and alert the emergency facility. Such patients can move into respiratory failure within minutes.

If the patient has less severe wheezing and a history of asthma, ask about medications. Sometimes patients take excessive amounts of certain inhalers (for example, over 12 to 14 puffs per day of beta agonists like albuterol). If this seems to be the case, review the situation with the clinician.

Sometimes patients are reluctant to combine inhalers even if advised to do so. Reassure them that it is perfectly acceptable practice to combine inhaled drugs of different types.

Do not recommend over-the-counter inhalers. These are weak bronchodilators. Better therapy is available under the clinician's supervision.

If a patient has mild wheezing and a history of mild asthma or a viral infection, a hot shower may help.

If the patient reports wheezing with exercise or exposure to cold air and he or she has previously been treated with an inhaled bronchodilator such as albuterol, suggest using the inhaler 10 to 15 minutes before exercising or going outside.

Patients who are wheezing and have symptoms of a lower respiratory infection (e.g., fever or cough with phlegm production) will nearly always need to be seen by a clinician. Tell the patient to call back if the symptoms worsen (e.g., increasing chest tightness or fever over 101.5°F) before the time of the appointment.

A
D
U
L
T

CHAPTER 62

Wounds

Marie-Eileen Onieal, MMHS, RN, CPNP

Wounds are one of the most common reasons people seek emergency treatment or advice. Any break in the integrity of the skin is cause for concern, because the skin provides the body with its prime defense against infection. Wounds can be divided into lacerations (jagged wounds or tears), abrasions (scrapes), and puncture wounds.

There are several important elements in assessing the severity of any wound:
- Whether bleeding can be controlled
- Whether sutures or other repair is needed
- Whether other structures have been damaged (e.g., a joint, the eye)
- Risk of infection
- Risk of tetanus

The location of the wound can be a clue to the mechanism of injury. Wounds around the genital area raise the suspicion of abuse, as do wounds to "out of reach" places on the body.

Gentle, firm pressure can stop the bleeding in a simple wound. Wounds in or around the mouth and at the forehead region appear to bleed profusely because of the rich blood supply to those areas. An initial blotting of the wound will aid in the assessment of the amount of bleeding.

Most superficial wounds or abrasions can be treated at home. Gentle washing with soap and warm water will remove foreign material and dead tissue, decreasing the risk of infection. If there is any question about the size of the wound or the need for sutures, the patient should be evaluated as soon as possible. Delay in evaluation and repair can increase the risk of infection. If the patient has multiple wounds or bleeding cannot be stopped within 10 minutes, the EMS system should be activated for transport to the nearest emergency facility.

Tetanus can infect any laceration or puncture wound, so it is important to determine the patient's tetanus immunization status. Abrasions are not tetanus-prone wounds. Tetanus immunization is advised:

- If it is more than 10 years since the last shot.
- If it is more than 5 years since the last shot and the wound is dirty or deep.
- If the person has not completed a full series of tetanus immunization.
- If the person has not been immunized at all. The series should be started right away and arrangements made for completion.

Redness, warmth, swelling, and drainage characterize wound infection. Any wound or abrasion that begins to show signs of infection should be evaluated as soon as possible.

LACERATIONS AND ABRASIONS

Question	To See Clinician If . . .	When
1. Patient's name, age, telephone number		
2. Is the wound bleeding now? Is the bleeding steady or pulsating?	Bleeding will not stop, especially if pulsating.	EMS
3. How and when did the injury occur?	Wound is dirty or involves force (machinery, power tools, crush injury).	2
4. Are you taking any medications? Do you have any bleeding disorders or other illnesses?	Patient is taking blood thinners (anticoagulants) or has anemia, hemophilia, or diabetes.	2
5. Is the wound gaping or deep?	Any evidence of depth or inability to close the wound (may require stitches).	2
6. Is any foreign body visible in the wound, or is a foreign body possible?	Yes, foreign body visible or possible.	2
7. Where is the laceration?	Over a joint, near or on the eye, on the genitals, in the mouth, or on the face.	2
8. When was your last tetanus shot?	Clean wound: more than 10 years ago. Dirty or deep wound: more than 5 years ago.	8

EMS = Activate EMS SYSTEM   24-72 = Appointment within 3 days

2 = See ASAP (within 1–2 hours)   72+ = Appointment in 4 days or more

8 = See same day

High priority items appear in color.

ADVICE

To stop bleeding, apply direct, firm pressure to the wound. If the patient is advised to go to the office or emergency facility, bleeding should be controlled while en route by applying firm pressure with a clean, dry cloth.

If the patient will not be coming immediately to the office or other care facility, the wound should be washed thoroughly:

- Flush with cool to warm running tap water. If the area cannot be put under the faucet, flush by pouring water over the area.
- Use a soft cloth to gently scrub with soap and water. Rinse thoroughly.
- Apply an antiseptic, like Polysporin, and cover with a Band-Aid or sterile gauze. Use a non-stick dressing for large abrasions.
- Inspect daily for any signs of infection, such as redness, warmth, swelling, or drainage. If these signs appear, call back immediately.

ADULT

233

TRAINING AND EVALUATING TELEPHONE STAFF

CHAPTER 63

A Four-Step Approach to Improving Telephone Service

Harvey P. Katz, MD

Telephone service, especially telephone triage, can be improved by taking a four-step approach that focuses on systems, policies, and people:

1. Monitor the existing telephone system with measurements (see Chapter 2) and analyze its strengths and weaknesses.
2. Train staff members by study of written materials, with clinician supervision.
3. Train staff members by observation of senior staff.
4. Regularly evaluate staff members' skills.

Step One: Monitor and Analyze the Existing Telephone System

Objectives

1. To analyze the current telephone system in a detailed, descriptive fashion, including the number of calls by hour and day of week, and time to answer. The focus should be on predicting the busiest hours so staffing levels can be increased at those times and planning staffing and other approaches to reduce volume and smooth out peaks wherever appropriate.
2. To evaluate the telephone behavior of staff members, service targets, and the current training program.

Methods

1. Use computer software (automatic call distribution, ACD) or a manual telephone encounter form to collect the important telephone data (total number of calls hourly and at peak times, number of calls for advice versus administrative or appointment information, number of referrals, and number of same-day appointments versus home management advice). Automated measurements, as discussed in Chapter 2, are recommended.
2. Clinicians and other supervisors should use a double headset to listen to the way support staff are answering the telephone and talking to patients.
3. Supervisors should call the office to evaluate the number of rings and the time it takes before the phone is answered, whether and how they were put on "hold," and how they were greeted.
4. Evaluate whether an adequate number of staff members are being deployed at peak times.
5. Ask a representative of the telephone company to observe the telephone behavior of office personnel and the mechanics of the present system and to make recommendations for improvement. This service is usually free.

Step Two: Train Staff Members by Study of Written Materials

Objectives

1. After study of training material, staff members should be able to obtain a relevant medical history and distinguish between:
   - A true emergency
   - Problems that can be safely managed at home
   - Problems that require an appointment
2. For problems that require an appointment, staff members should be able to determine when the appointment is needed:
   - Immediately—activate EMS/911 for emergency situations
   - As soon as possible—within 2 hours
   - Same day—within 8 hours
   - Future appointment—within 3 days
   - Future appointment—in 4 days or more
3. Staff members should be able to present home management advice for specific symptoms accurately, safely, and efficiently.
4. Staff members should be aware of the differences between patient evaluations by telephone and those carried out face to face and should know how to avoid potential pitfalls and errors (see Chapter 5).
5. Staff members should understand that the voice creates an image of the practice and recognize the value of professional telephone behavior to the medical program (see Chapter 4).

Methods

1. Staff members should study this book and other references as needed.
2. Telephone role playing, in which one member of the support staff plays the patient and the other plays the telephone assistant, should be incorporated into team meetings. The case scenarios described in Chapter 64 can be used in combination with those created by the staff from actual cases. Live taping of encounters can be a powerful learning tool; always inform patients beforehand that the conversation is being taped.

3. Regular office or team meetings should include lectures and discussions about specific disease entities and management techniques.

Step Three: Train Staff Members by Observation of Senior Staff

Objectives

1. To develop staff expertise in history taking, improving the ability to differentiate between problems that need appointments and those that can be handled safely with home management advice
2. To learn how to schedule appointments and keep pace with heavy volume
3. To learn how to respond to acute emergency situations
4. To learn how to manage upset or angry patients
5. To become fully informed about the management of administrative matters, including:
   - Prescription refills
   - Requests for laboratory results
   - Referrals
   - Health education information, such as immunization schedules and preventive medicine advice, as prescribed by the practice

Methods

1. All new staff members should spend approximately 24 hours (over a period of 2 months) directly observing an experienced senior staff member, listening to telephone conversations on a double headset adjusted for simultaneous listening only.
2. Illustrative cases and actual telephone encounters should be discussed with the supervising clinician.

Step Four: Regularly Evaluate Staff Members' Skills

Objectives

1. To evaluate the telephone assistants' ability to distinguish between emergency situations, problems that need appointments, and problems that can be safely managed at home and to handle each situation appropriately
2. To improve knowledge and skill by constructive dialogue
3. To encourage outside reading and other study in areas recommended by the supervising clinician

Methods

1. Each telephone assistant should have a 1-hour appointment to meet with each clinician in the health care team or medical practice.
2. Topics (two or three each) should be divided among the clinicians and distributed in advance to the telephone assistant in preparation for the meeting.
3. Role playing should be incorporated into the evaluation using the audit forms from Chapter 64 as examples. The Assessment Summary Form (see Table 64–1) can be used to record and communicate the results of this exercise.
4. Tapes of actual telephone scenarios, or video scripts if they are available, should be used as springboards for discussion.
5. Strong points should be congratulated, and further study assigned in areas needing improvement (see Appendix B).

CHAPTER 64

∎∎∎∎∎∎∎∎∎∎∎∎
∎
∎
∎
∎

Case Studies for Role-Playing

One of the major objectives of this book is to help with the evaluation of telephone personnel. A basic "Audit Form" has been designed to assess whether key questions are being asked when patients call with a problem. This chapter presents brief case studies of telephone calls that concern a few important pediatric and adult symptoms from those covered in Sections Three and Four and includes a list of the types of questions that a skilled telephone assistant would be expected to ask each caller. These scenarios can be used for role-playing sessions with clinicians, or the lists can be used to evaluate real conversations between triage staff and patients. (Serious consideration should be given to the evaluation of randomly selected live tapes.) In this way, the supervising health professional can engage the telephone assistant in educational dialogue. The questions on each Audit Form are similar to the questions in each set of Telephone Decision Guidelines in Sections Three and Four, so if no Audit Form has been provided for a specific situation, the supervising clinician can use the telephone guidelines as a basis for training or quality control for the triage staff, following the pattern of the cases and forms in this chapter.

This training and evaluation process should take place with all new personnel and should be repeated periodically with the more senior staff members so that the clinician can readily evaluate the capabilities and judgment being exercised on the telephone. The Assessment Summary Form (Table 64–1) can be used to record and communicate the results of this exercise. The atmosphere initially might be somewhat inhibited, but with gentle encouragement staff members quickly relax, particularly when the constructive and educational objective of the audit exercise is emphasized, rather than just the "quiz" aspect. Importantly, these sessions also enable the clinician to impart his or her own individual approach to the evaluation of specific illnesses. The sessions also will stimulate the telephone assistant by providing continuing medical education and a sense of teamwork and bonding with clinicians and other staff members.

To stimulate additional study, a few additional resources about each topic are listed in Appendix B at the end of the book, each one annotated to point out its value and relevance. Staff members should be encouraged to consult these resources to deepen or update their knowledge.

TABLE 64-1   Assessment Summary Form for Staff Members

This generic assessment form helps evaluate telephone management performance. It should be used to supplement each of the symptom-specific Audit Forms in Chapter 64 or for similar evaluations of other scenarios. Both strengths and weaknesses should be highlighted.

1. Was there a four-part verbal handshake (greeting, name, practice or department, and offer to help)?

2. Was the telephone style assertive, professional, informed, and caring?

3. Were closed- and open-ended questions used appropriately?

4. Was the decision to advise home management or an office appointment appropriate in this instance? If a visit was advised, was the timing of the visit appropriate (emergency, as soon as possible, same day, future appointment)? If this was an emergency scenario, was it accurately identified and managed as such?

5. Were the key, relevant questions asked in obtaining the history?

6. If not, what other questions should have been asked to help evaluate the needs in this patient encounter?

7. Were the instructions given to this patient clear, concise, and accurate?

8. Was the amount of time spent reaching closure appropriate to this problem?

(Continued)

TABLE 64–1 **Assessment Summary Form for Staff Members** *(Continued)*
9. What were the strengths exhibited in this telephone encounter?
10. Were there areas in the telephone encounter that might be improved?
11. Are there any recommendations for further study or for additional practice?

AUDIT FORM

. . . .

ABDOMINAL PAIN (PEDIATRIC)

Mr. Turner calls about his 9-year-old son, who has a stomachache. He was called by the school to come and pick Joseph up because the boy was complaining all morning that his stomach hurt and he vomited once in the health room. Mr. Turner is now home with Joseph and wants to know what to do.

Were the Following Items Noted?

1. Was there an appropriate identification and greeting?	Yes	No
2. Name, telephone number, age of patient?	Yes	No
3. Severity of pain?	Yes	No
4. Any trauma?	Yes	No
5. Location of pain?	Yes	No
6. Child acting ill or lethargic?	Yes	No
7. Any other symptoms?	Yes	No
• Fever?	Yes	No
• Vomiting?	Yes	No
• Diarrhea?	Yes	No
• Severe cough or difficulty breathing?	Yes	No
• Burning or frequency of urination?	Yes	No
• Constipation?	Yes	No
8. Duration of pain?	Yes	No
9. Is pain constant or intermittent?	Yes	No
10. Is pain getting better, worse, or about the same?	Yes	No
11. Family members ill with similar symptoms?	Yes	No
12. Any chronic medical condition?	Yes	No
13. Has child been seen for this problem in the past?	Yes	No

Evaluation: Use Assessment Summary Form (Table 64–1) on pages 239–240.

AUDIT FORM
. . . .
CROUP (PEDIATRIC)

A snowstorm has struck. It is early morning and people cannot get out of their homes. The staff has made it to the office, but the clinicians will be at the hospital all morning. Scott, the Alexanders' 3-year-old son, awoke this morning with a cough that sounded like a foghorn. He has had a mild cold for the past 3 days.

Were the Following Items Noted?

1. Was there an appropriate identification and greeting?	Yes	No
2. Name, telephone number, and age of child?	Yes	No
3. How long has barking cough been present?	Yes	No
4. Are lips bluish?	Yes	No
5. Drooling or difficulty in swallowing?	Yes	No
6. Has child choked or possibly gotten something stuck in throat?	Yes	No
7. Loud noise with each breath?	Yes	No
8. Does chest cave in as he breathes?	Yes	No
9. Fever or other symptoms (earache, sore throat, looks ill, pale, or frightened)?	Yes	No
10. Is child lethargic or refusing fluids?	Yes	No
11. Any chronic or serious medical conditions?	Yes	No

In answer to questions, Mrs. Alexander reports that Scott's temperature is 100.4°F. He is playful, alert, and in no distress. He is hoarse, but taking fluids well. Home advice should have been given with instructions to call back if his condition worsened. At 10:00 A.M., Mrs. Alexander calls back and reports that Scott suddenly is worse. His lips have turned blue and he is agitated.

1. Does the advice change to activating the emergency medical system (EMS/911)?	Yes	No

Evaluation: Use Assessment Summary Form (Table 64–1) on pages 239–240.

AUDIT FORM
. . . .

DIARRHEA (PEDIATRIC)

The first call of the morning comes from a parent who reports that his 3-year-old daughter has had loose stools for the past day, and now her bowel movement is "pure water."

Were the Following Items Noted?

1. Was there an appropriate identification and greeting?   Yes   No

2. Name, telephone number, and age of child?   Yes   No

3. How many bowel movements in past 12 to 24 hours?   Yes   No

4. Signs of dehydration (listless, dry tongue and inner cheek, no tears   Yes   No
   when crying, sunken eyeballs, no urine for 8 to 10 hours)?

5. Blood or mucus in the stool?   Yes   No

6. Does child appear ill?   Yes   No

7. Any abdominal pain?   Yes   No

8. Other symptoms? Fever?   Yes   No
   - Jack-knifing knees?   Yes   No
   - Earache?   Yes   No
   - Vomiting?   Yes   No
   - Hard, fast breathing?   Yes   No

9. How long has child had diarrhea?   Yes   No

10. Medications?   Yes   No

11. Usual state of health?   Yes   No

12. On clear liquid diet? How long?   Yes   No

Evaluation: Use Assessment Summary Form (Table 64–1) on pages 239–240.

AUDIT FORM
. . . .

FEVER (PEDIATRIC)

Ms. Jefferson calls to report that, on awakening this morning, her 4-year-old son Dwight appeared lethargic and glassy-eyed. She took his temperature and it was 102°F, orally.

Were the Following Items Noted?

1. Was there an appropriate identification and greeting?   Yes   No

2. Name, telephone number, and age of child?   Yes   No

3. Does child appear particularly ill, irritable, or lethargic?   Yes   No

4. Has child ever had a convulsion?   Yes   No

5. Duration of fever? Temperature?   Yes   No

6. Complete review of systems?
   - CNS—headache out of proportion to fever? Stiff neck?   Yes   No
   - Respiratory—breathing difficulty, rapid breathing?   Yes   No
   - Skin—rash?   Yes   No
   - GU—burning or frequency of urination?   Yes   No
   - ENT—cough, sneezing, sore throat, earache?   Yes   No
   - GI—vomiting or diarrhea?   Yes   No

7. Any other medical condition?   Yes   No

8. Medicine given (dose and frequency)?   Yes   No

Evaluation: Use Assessment Summary Form (Table 64–1) on pages 239–240.

ALLERGIC REACTIONS AND ANAPHYLAXIS (ADULT)

A 44-year-old woman had been sitting in her back yard. She had just completed her dinner and had taken her evening medications. At approximately 6:30 P.M., she experienced the abrupt onset of generalized itching and hives. Within minutes, she also noted hoarseness, difficulty in swallowing, and stridor.

Were the Following Items Noted?

1. Was there an appropriate identification and greeting?   Yes   No

2. Name, telephone number, and characteristics of patient?   Yes   No

3. Progression of symptoms: Hives and swelling, respiratory distress,   Yes   No
   stridor or wheezing, dysphagia, nausea and vomiting, faintness or
   loss of consciousness?

4. Has anaphylaxis occurred in the past and, if so, how severe?   Yes   No

5. Is the patient alone?   Yes   No

6. Has an epinephrine auto-injector (e.g., EpiPen) previously been   Yes   No
   prescribed and administered?

7. What are the suspected causes?   Yes   No

8. Was the patient stung?   Yes   No

9. What medications had been taken at the time of this reaction?   Yes   No

10. What foods were eaten at the evening meal?   Yes   No

11. Does the patient have any cardiovascular or CNS disease?   Yes   No

12. Is the patient taking a beta blocker (including ocular) or ACE inhibitor? Yes   No

13. Is the patient taking an MAO inhibitor or tricyclic antidepressant? Yes   No

Evaluation: Use Assessment Summary Form (Table 64–1) on pages 239–240.

AUDIT FORM
. . . .
BACK PAIN (ADULT)

Mr. Banks, a 38-year-old construction worker, calls because of severe pain in his low back, which began when he picked up a heavy object an hour ago. He says the pain goes all the way down the back of his leg and there is some tingling in his foot.

Were the Following Items Noted?

1. Was there an appropriate identification and greeting?   Yes   No

2. Name, telephone number, and characteristics of patient?   Yes   No

3. Urinary incontinence?   Yes   No

4. Weakness or numbness in legs?   Yes   No

5. History of cancer?   Yes   No

6. Fever?   Yes   No

7. Pain running down back of thigh?   Yes   No

8. Is patient alarmed?   Yes   No

Evaluation: Use Assessment Summary Form (Table 64–1) on pages 239–240.

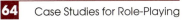

AUDIT FORM

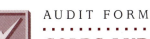

COLDS AND FLU (ADULT)

A 51-year-old man complains of cough productive of yellow-green sputum. The cough keeps him up at night. He smoked one pack of cigarettes per day for 20 years, stopping 10 years ago.

Were the Following Items Noted?

1. Was there an appropriate identification and greeting?	Yes	No
2. Name, phone number, and characteristics of patient?	Yes	No
3. Is there shortness of breath or chest pain?	Yes	No
4. Is there fever?	Yes	No
5. Has the patient coughed up dark or bloody sputum?	Yes	No
6. Does patient have other serious medical problems?	Yes	No
7. Duration of cough? Improving?	Yes	No

Evaluation: Use Assessment Summary Form (Table 64–1) on pages 239–240.

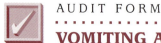

A U D I T   F O R M

· ·

VOMITING AND NAUSEA (ADULT)

Mrs. Johnson, a 32-year-old woman, calls to report that she has been "throwing up." She has had some watery diarrhea as well. Her 9-year-old son has similar symptoms.

Were the Following Items Noted?

1. Was there an appropriate identification and greeting?	Yes	No
2. Name, telephone number, and characteristics of patient?	Yes	No
3. What did the vomit contents look like?	Yes	No
4. Was there any head injury?	Yes	No
5. Is there abdominal pain?	Yes	No
6. Is there any fever?	Yes	No
7. Is there a history of abdominal surgery?	Yes	No
8. Is there lightheadedness?	Yes	No
9. Is the urine dark yellow?	Yes	No
10. Is there skin tenting?	Yes	No
11. Has urine volume or frequency decreased?	Yes	No
12. Is concentration poor or slow?	Yes	No
13. Is mouth dry?	Yes	No
14. Has patient been unable to take anything by mouth for more than a day?	Yes	No
15. Could patient be pregnant?	Yes	No
16. Was patient exposed to spoiled food?	Yes	No
17. Are the stools loose?	Yes	No
18. Is patient taking any new medications?	Yes	No
19. Does patient have any major medical illnesses?	Yes	No
20. How is the child? Has his pediatrician been notified?	Yes	No

Evaluation: Use Assessment Summary Form (Table 64–1) on pages 239–240.

APPENDIX A

A Patient's Guide to Effective Use of the Telephone

Harvey P. Katz, MD

When you select a primary care clinician (pediatrician, family practitioner, internist, nurse practitioner, or physician assistant), a patient-clinician team is formed. As a team member, you have certain responsibilities. The more actively you carry out your responsibilities, the more effectively the telephone will work for both you and your clinician. Telephone communication with the clinician and the office staff, and ultimately the quality of care that you receive, will be improved immeasurably if you actively try to:

- Be informed
- Be descriptive
- Be assertive
- Be understanding

Be Informed

- Learn about the office phone system, such as the best hours to call for nonurgent questions such as advice, billing, and routine prescription refills. Some practices have specific call-in times. Know whether your office has them, and observe them. You can save time by not calling during peak telephone hours for routine appointments. Peak time should be reserved for acute and urgent problems that require immediate advice or an appointment the same day. Peak hours for practices treating adults usually occur in the early morning and at noon. Peak hours for practices treating children include early mornings and late afternoons when children return home from school. The day after a 3-day weekend is particularly busy for all offices.
- Ask questions and always have a notepad and pen handy so that you can write down any instructions you receive. If you have one, keep your medical record number handy.
- Know who answers the phone—Are you speaking with a nurse or non-nurse?
- Know what other professionals work in the office: doctors, physician assistants, nurse practitioners? What is the role of each of these people?
- Under what circumstances might you use the hospital emergency room?
- Many large groups and HMOs have a Website, which may be an excellent source of information about the group practice, including biographies and profiles of the clinicians with whom you will be dealing.

Be Descriptive

- When you call the office, describe the problem briefly and objectively. Try to present an accurate history with the relevant details: "My daughter, Susan, is 6 years old and has had a loose chest cough and fever for the past 5 days. I have been giving her Tylenol every 4 hours with lots of fluids but it is not working. Today she has a temperature of 103°F and is much worse. I would like to bring her in to see a doctor this morning." This description is much more effective than "Susan isn't feeling well today and feels warm. I'm not sure what to do."

Be Assertive

- If you really want to speak to your clinician rather than the nurse, be direct. Let the office nurse or appointment secretary know that you want to speak to your clinician, the nature of problem and when you would like a call-back. "This is Charles Jones. I would like to speak to my primary physician, Dr. Ross, about my continuing sore throat. He saw me yesterday. If he is not there, please have him call me this afternoon between 3 and 5 P.M." Be brief and to the point.
- If you feel the situation is an emergency, tell the person answering the phone (either in the office or an answering service) that "this is an emergency" in order to avoid delay.
- If you are placed on "hold" before you get a chance to say anything, call back and object. This is an unsafe situation because you might be reporting an emergency. Always let the doctor or office supervisor know if you are dissatisfied about any aspect of the telephone system. A responsive practice will appreciate the constructive feedback and try to improve.
- If you want an appointment, say so. Don't be equivocal or be talked out of one if you want to be seen.

Be Understanding

- If you are "on hold" for longer than usual, recognize that calls about emergencies will be given highest priority while others must wait.
- If an appointment time that's suggested conflicts with a personal commitment, try to rearrange your schedule. This will allow your clinician to better serve your needs. Your flexibility in scheduling appointments will be appreciated.

Be Prepared

- As mentioned above, always have a pencil and paper next to the telephone.
- For illnesses that may involve a fever, take the temperature before you call. You'll save time.
- Keep frequently used telephone numbers near your telephone: physician, hospital emergency room, poison control center, 24-hour pharmacy, HMO or insurance company customer service and billing office.
- Have a medicine chest well stocked with up-to-date supplies. When your clinician or office nurse gives home treatment advice, it saves valuable time to have the appropriate medication and equipment on hand.

TABLE A-1 **Basic Contents of the Well-Stocked Medicine Cabinet**

Over-the-Counter Medication

Acetaminophen and/or ibuprofen, pediatric and adult, to reduce fever and relieve pain
Aspirin for adults (not to be given to children because of link to Reye's syndrome)
Antacid
Antihistamine
Antidiarrheal (for adults and teenagers)
Cough medication with non-narcotic cough suppressant
Decongestant
Syrup of ipecac (1-ounce bottle) to induce vomiting (only if advised by poison control or
  physician)
Saline nose drops and bulb syringe for young infants
1% hydrocortisone cream
Calamine lotion
Antibiotic ointment
Vaseline

Equipment and First Aid Kit

Band-Aids and adhesive tape
2- and 4-inch sterile gauze pads
Q-tips
Sterile cotton balls
Thermometer
Butterfly Band-Aid or steristrips (for minor lacerations)
Calibrated medicine spoon
Disposable nonlatex gloves
Tweezers
Blunt bandage scissors
Rubbing alcohol

Home Health Center

A well-stocked medicine cabinet should contain prescription medication that is current (as a rule, drugs that are less than 1 year old), selected over-the-counter medications for treating minor illness and injuries, and a first aid tool kit (Table A-1). If family members have chronic illnesses, more specialized equipment to round out the home health center may include items such as a blood pressure cuff for a patient with high blood pressure, a glucose monitor for a diabetic patient, or a peak flow meter for asthma monitoring.

Medicine cabinets frequently are themselves in need of treatment. Contrary to tradition, the bathroom is not the best location for your medicines. The increased moisture and heat cause medications to deteriorate. Select a dry, cool, and dark place such as an easily accessed shelf in a linen closet. The closet should be locked if children live in or visit the home.

Once a year, clean out and update the cabinet. Carefully discard all expired or unused prescription and over-the counter medications.

Flush outdated medication down the toilet. Never throw medicine or medical equipment in a wastebasket where young children or teens are likely to find it.

APPENDIX B

Suggestions for Further Study

THE TELEPHONE IN THE PRIMARY HEALTH CARE PRACTICE

Chapter 1: The Role of the Telephone in Medical Care— An Overview

Blankenship, JC: The telephone booth: A worthwhile stop along the information superhighway. Am J Med 108:592–593, 2000.
> *This paper discusses the many documented ways in which the quality of patient care has been improved by telephone medicine, which is a powerful tool in the practice of medicine.*

Katz, HP: Quality of telephone medicine. HMO Practice 4:137–141, 1990.
> *The ingredients necessary for a successful telephone medicine program in office practice are outlined. The importance of training to prepare staff for their critical role in telephone triage is stressed.*

Smith, K: Telephone health care: It's more than just a phone call. Pediatric Nursing 25:423–429, 1999.
> *This article calls attention to the fact that there is more to telephone medicine than answering the phone. It discusses the unique skills and knowledge (referred to by some as "telehealth") and telephone competencies needed for success in telephone health care.*

Chapter 2: Organizing an Office Telephone Care System

Bergeron, BP: Get in with the e-crowd. Digital Doc 107:31–34, 2000.
> *Outlines some ways to keep e-mail in check in order to serve your medical practice.*

Elnicki, DM, et al: Telephone medicine for internists. JGIM 15:337–343, 2000.
> *Comprehensive literature review of the role of the telephone in primary care internal medicine. The paper describes telephone utilization and makes some comparisons to other specialties.*

Friedman, RH: Automated telephone conversations to assess health behavior and deliver behavioral interventions. Journal of Medical Systems 22:95–101, 1998.
> *Good description of the technology, history, and practical application of telephone-linked-care (TLC) to behavioral interventions in primary care.*

Glowniak, J: History, structure, and function of the Internet. Seminars in Nuclear Medicine 28:135–144, 1998.
> *Historical article describing the development of the Internet over the past 30 to 40 years to its current place at the forefront of telecommunications in medicine.*

Kane, B, and Sands, DZ, for the AMIA Internet Working Group, Task Force on Guidelines for the Use of Clinic-Patient Electronic Mail: Guidelines for the clinical use of electronic mail with patients. JAMIA 5:104–111, 1998.
> *A white paper that is "must reading" for those thinking about using e-mail in their practice. General discussion and guidelines address the issues of effective interaction between clinician and patient and the need for medicolegal prudence.*

Mandl, KD, et al: Electronic patient-physician communication: Problems and promise. Annals of Internal Medicine 129:495–500, 1998.

> *Excellent, balanced discussion of the pros and cons of e-mail in medical practice provides a research agenda to evaluate this technology before it becomes widespread.*

Chapter 3: Medicolegal Issues in Telephone Medicine

Katz, HP: Malpractice, meningitis, and the telephone. Pediatric Annals 20:85–89, 1992.

> *Details of real-life malpractice suit, one of the first to focus on the role of the triage nurse in the outcome of a child with meningitis.*

Telephones and electronic technology (Questions 31–39). In 100 Questions about Health Care Risk Management. Risk Management Foundation of the Harvard Medical Institutions, Cambridge, MA, 1996, pp 31–39.

> *Common themes for medicolegal question, with answers compiled by a risk management foundation in the course of their years of work in the field.*

Wick, WR, and Katz, HP: Telephone contacts and counseling. In American College of Legal Medicine (ed): Legal Medicine, ed 3. Mosby–Year Book, St. Louis, 1995, pp 343–350.

> *Telephone medicine as a medicolegal risk is discussed from the legal point of view. Cases that have focused on the telephone as the major reason for the claim are included, along with the steps required to reduce risk in primary care practice.*

TELEPHONE SKILLS IN PRIMARY HEALTH CARE

Chapter 4: The Art of Telephone Medicine

Wheeler, SQ: Telephone Triage, Theory, Practice and Protocol Development. Delmar Publishers, Albany, NY, 1993, pp 43–72.

> *Good discussion of communication theory, skills, and style.*

Chapter 5: The Medical History

Coulehan, JL, and Block, MR: The Medical Interview: Mastering Skills for Clinical Practice, ed 4. FA Davis, Philadelphia, 2001.

> *An excellent introduction to history-taking for all health care professionals, with an emphasis on building a satisfactory clinician-patient relationship.*

Chapter 6: Prescribing Medication Over the Telephone

2000 PDR for Nonprescription Drugs and Dietary Supplements (new edition available annually). Medical Economics, Montvale, NJ.

> *Authoritative guide to the use of the most commonly used OTC medications, with FDA-approved descriptions. New edition includes section on vitamins, herbs, and dietary supplements.*

Berlin, CM, Jr: Acetaminophen and ibuprofen: Instructing parents on dosing. Contemporary Pediatrics (Supplement), September 1999, pp 3–11.

> *Excellent summary of how to use the two most common antifever medications correctly.*

OTC Products. In Pharmacy Times, Supplement, Pharmacy Times, Westbury, NY, Sept. 1999.

> *The pharmaceutical industry's annual summary of OTC use and trends based on sales data from across the United States. A summary of the most popular over-the-counter products recommended by pharmacists.*

SYMPTOMS IN CHILDREN

Chapter 8: Abdominal Pain

Boyle, J: Recurrent abdominal pain: An update. Pediatrics in Review 18:310–320, 1997.

> *Excellent discussion of differential diagnosis. Article highlights "red flags" that may differentiate organic disease from functional disorders.*

DiPalma, AM, and DiPalma, JA: Recurrent abdominal pain and lactose maldigestion in school-aged children. Gastroenterology Nursing 20:180–183, 1997.
> *This review focuses on the diagnosis and management of lactose intolerance as an important cause of recurrent abdominal pain in children.*

Montgomery, D, and Horman, M: Acute abdominal pain: A challenge for the practitioner. Journal of Pediatric Health Care 12:157–159, 1998.
> *Differential diagnosis, clinical presentation, laboratory studies, and management of acute abdominal pain and its evaluation.*

Chapter 9: Animal Bites

American Academy of Pediatrics, Committee on Infectious Diseases: Bite wounds. 1997 Red Book, ed 24. American Academy of Pediatrics, Elk Grove Village, IL, pp 122–126.
> *Authoritative recommendations for prophylactic management and antimicrobial treatment for animal bite wounds.*

Connelly, KP: Advising families about pets. Contemporary Pediatrics 14:77–78, 1997.
> *This is a guide for parents, with procedures for introducing a baby to a dog.*

Tulan, DA, et al: Bacteriologic analysis of infected dog and cat bites. N Engl J Med 340:85–92, 1996.
> *Prospective study at 18 emergency departments to define bacteria from dog and cat bites uncovered organisms not previously recognized as introduced by bite wounds. Rationale for treatment recommendations discussed.*

Chapter 10: Asthma

Newson, T, and McKenzie, S: Cough and asthma in children. Pediatric Annals 25:156–8, 161, 1996.
> *Article points out the difficulty in diagnosing asthma and discusses an approach to suspecting asthma in patients with chronic cough.*

Plaut, TF: One Minute Asthma: What You Need to Know, ed 3. Pedipress, Amherst, MA, 1996.
> *What you need to know about asthma in practical, easily understood directions appropriate for both parents and clinicians.*

Practical Guide for the Diagnosis and Management of Asthma. National Asthma Education and Prevention Program: Expert Panel Report No. 2. National Institutes of Health Publication, No. A7-4053, October 1997.
> *Comprehensive and authoritative guide based on an expert panel convened to describe how primary care clinicians can improve asthma care. Major recommendations are nicely summarized.*

Torda, W: Asthma. In Dershewitz, RA (ed): Ambulatory Pediatric Care, ed 3. Lippincott-Raven, Philadelphia, 1999, pp 329–337.
> *Excellent, concise discussion of clinical presentation, workup, and treatment. Detailed recommendations for pharmacologic treatment are based on severity of asthma.*

Chapter 11: Burns and Sunburn

Allwood, JS: The primary care management of burns. Nurse Practitioner 20:77–79, 1995.
> *The physiologic alterations with burns are presented as the basis for assessment and treatment.*

Clayton, MC, and Solem, LD: No ice, no butter. Advice on management of burns for primary care physicians. Postgraduate Medicine 97:151–155, 1995.
> *The authors review types of burns and describe those that are easily treated versus those that should be referred to a burn center.*

Heffernan, AE, and O'Sullivan, A: Pediatric sun exposure. Nurse Practitioner 23:67–68, 1998.
> *Appropriate use of sunscreen can reduce risk of skin cancer. Prevention is emphasized, because the risk of malignant melanoma may double if severe sunburn occurs during childhood.*

Chapter 12: Colds

Clemens, CS, et al: Is an antihistamine-decongestant (ADC) combination effective in temporarily relieving symptoms of the common cold in preschool children? Journal of Pediatrics 130:463–466, 1997.
> *ADC was equivalent to placebo in providing temporary relief but did cause significant drowsiness as a significant side effect.*

MacKnin, ML, et al: Zinc lozenges for treating the common cold in children. JAMA 279:1962–1967, 1998.
Zinc gluconate lozenges caused more adverse side effects, such as nausea and diarrhea, and were ineffective in relieving cold symptoms in children and adolescents.

NyQuist, AC, et al: Antibiotic prescribing for children with colds, upper respiratory tract infections, and bronchitis. JAMA 279:875–877, 1998.
A study of 531 pediatric office visits, which confirmed that patients with colds, URIs, and bronchitis typically do not benefit from antibiotic treatment.

Chapter 13: Constipation

Baker, SS, et al: Constipation in infants and children. A medical position statement of the North American Society for Pediatric Gastroenterology and Nutrition. Journal of Pediatric Gastroenterology and Nutrition 29:612–626, 1999.
Clinical guidelines for managing constipation, written for primary care clinicians and covering evaluation, treatment, and indications for referral to a pediatric gastroenterologist.

Loening-Baucke, V: Chronic constipation in children. Gastroenterology 105:1557–1564, 1993.
Excellent review article describing how to evaluate and treat constipation.

Pettei, MJ: Constipation and encopresis. In Gellis, S, and Kagan, B (eds): Current Pediatric Therapy, ed 15. WB Saunders, Philadelphia, 1996, pp 269–271.
Importance of history and physical examination in the early recognition of chronic problems. Preventive dietary measures are stressed.

Chapter 14: Croup

Folland, DS: Treatment of croup. Sending home an improved child and relieved parents. Postgraduate Medicine 101:271–273, 277–278, 1997.
Most children with croup, the most common cause of upper airway obstruction in childhood, can be treated effectively as outpatients. This paper describes both emergency room treatment and home management.

Geelhoed, GC: Croup. Pediatric Pulmonology 23:370–374, 1997.
This article discusses the current management of croup, emphasizing the changes in treatment over the last several years. The use of steroids is highlighted.

Chapter 15: Diarrhea

Kneepkens, CM, and Hoekstra, JH: Chronic nonspecific diarrhea of childhood: Pathophysiology and management. Pediatric Clinics of North America 43:375–390, 1996.
Comprehensive discussion of toddler's diarrhea, or chronic nonspecific diarrhea of childhood, as primarily a gut-motility disorder. Management by normalization of the child's diet is stressed.

Lifschitz, CH: Treatment of acute diarrhea in children. Current Opinion in Pediatrics 9:498–501, 1997.
Two thorough papers chronicle recent publications on gastroenteritis and summarize the recommendations of the American Academy of Pediatrics. Early refeeding and oral rehydration are highlighted.

Lleung, AK, and Robson, WL: Evaluating the child with chronic diarrhea. American Family Physician 53:635–643, 1996.
This paper relates the causes of diarrhea to age of onset. Excellent and comprehensive review of differential diagnosis.

Chapter 16: Earache

Byington, CL: The diagnosis and management of otitis media with effusion (OME). Pediatric Annals 27:96–100, 1998.
Discusses the controversy about the surgical versus medical management of OME.

Conrad, DA: Should acute otitis media ever be treated with antibiotics? Pediatric Annals 27:66–74, 1998.
Reviews studies comparing antibacterial treatment to nonantibiotic therapy and recommends guidelines for those cases of otitis media in which antimicrobial therapy might be withheld or delayed.

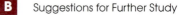

Heikkinen, T, and Ruuskanen, O: Otitis media. Current Opinion in Pediatrics 10:9–12, 1998.
This review article challenges the common practice of using antimicrobial prophylaxis for the prevention of otitis media.

Karver, SB: Otitis media. Primary Care; Clinics in Office Practice 25:619–632, 1998.
This paper clarifies the definitions of otitis media, acute otitis, and otitis with effusion and discusses the emergence of antimicrobial resistance to antibiotic treatment.

Chapter 17: Eye Infection and Inflammation

Ruppert, SD: Differential diagnosis of pediatric conjunctivitis (red eye). Nurse Practitioner 21:15–18, 1996.
This paper emphasizes accurate diagnosis of the red eye and prompt treatment of the underlying cause.

Wald, ER: Conjunctivitis in infants and children. Pediatric Infectious Disease Journal 16(2 suppl):17–20, 1997.
Excellent review of the causes and optimal treatment of conjunctivitis. H. influenzae is the most common cause of the combined "Conjunctivitis–Otitis" syndrome.

Yetman, RJ, and Coody, DK: Conjunctivitis: A practice guideline. Journal of Pediatric Health Care 11:238–241, 1997.
Excellent clinical guideline that includes definition, differential diagnosis of types of infection, rational approach to treatment based on etiology, and indications for referral.

Chapter 18: Fever

Bonadio, WA: The history and physical assessment of the febrile infant. Pediatric Clinics of North America 45:65–77, 1998.
This paper discusses the use of the Young Infant Observation Scale and the Yale Observation Scale as an effective way to classify the severity of illness of infants with fever.

Chinnock, R, et al: Hot tots: Current approach to the young febrile infant. Comprehensive Therapy 21:109–114, 1995.
This article presents an approach to identifying infants who can be managed safely as outpatients.

McCarthy PL, et al: Fever without apparent source on clinical examination, infectious disease, and lower respiratory infections in children. Current Opinion in Pediatrics 10:101–116, 1998.
This is an excellent review of the literature and focuses on those childhood infectious diseases that are commonly seen in office practice.

Chapter 19: Headaches

Gladstein, J: Headaches: The pediatrician's perspective. Seminars in Pediatric Neurology 2(2):119–126, 1995.
The role of the primary care physician is discussed. The article reviews the most common physical causes of headache, including infections, trauma, hypertension, pseudotumor cerebri, and ocular disorders.

Holder, EW, et al: Recurrent pediatric headaches: Assessment and intervention. Journal of Development and Behavioral Pediatrics 19(2):109–116, 1998.
A broad overview of the diagnosis and causes of recurrent headache is presented. Drug treatment and behavioral management research are reviewed.

Scheller, JM: The history, epidemiology, and classification of headaches in childhood. Seminars in Pediatric Neurology 2:102–108, 1995.
This paper is a good review of the epidemiology and classification of headaches. Symptoms, prevalence, school absences, risk factors, and treatment are discussed.

Smith, MS: Comprehensive evaluation and treatment of recurrent pediatric headache. Pediatric Annals 24:453–457, 1995.
The importance of continuity of care and regular follow-up is stressed in the successful management of recurrent pediatric headaches.

Chapter 20: Head Injury

Cantu, RC: Head and spine injuries in youth sports. Clinics in Sports Medicine 14:517–532, 1995.
Epidemiology of sports-related injuries is reviewed, focusing on types of injury and outcome.

Johnson, DL, and Krishnamurthy, S: Severe pediatric head injury: Myth, magic and actual fact. Pediatric Neurosurgery 28:167–172, 1998.
Study comparing outcome in 4041 head-injured children with 14,789 adults from Level I trauma centers. Mortality rates were comparable.

Mansfield, RT: Head injuries in children and adults. Critical Care Clinics 13:611–628, 1997.
Review of injuries from motor vehicle related accidents with focus on neurological complications.

Chapter 21: Insect Bites and Stings

Anthony, G, Jr: Insect stings. In Gellis, S, and Kagan, B (eds): Current Pediatric Therapy, ed 15. WB Saunders, Philadelphia, 1996, pp 734–735.
Helpful summary of treatment of anaphylaxis and local reactions. Discussion of prevention, emergency kits, and venom immunotherapy is practical and concise.

Hebert, AA, and Carlton, SR: Getting bugs to bug off: A review of insect repellents. Contemporary Pediatrics 15:85–95, 1998.
Discussion of insect repellents that describes various products and offers advice on how to choose and use them safely. Stresses that DEET concentrations should be no greater than 10% in repellents used on children.

Chapter 22: Nosebleed

Guarisco, JL, and Graham, HD: Epistaxis in children: Causes, diagnosis, and treatment. Ear, Nose, and Throat Journal 68:522–532, 1989.
Comprehensive discussion including causes and various treatment options.

McDonald, TJ: Nosebleed in children. Background and techniques to stop the flow. Postgraduate Medicine 81:217–224, 1987.
Practical review of causes and techniques for the primary care clinician.

Roberson, DW: Epistaxis. In Dershewitz, RA (ed): Ambulatory Pediatric Care, ed 3. Lippincott-Raven, Philadelphia, 1999, pp 475–477.
Management of acute and recurrent episodes of nosebleed, with indications of referral to specialist.

Chapter 23: Poisoning

American Academy of Pediatrics, Committee on Injury and Poison Prevention: Handbook of Common Poisonings in Children, ed 3. American Academy of Pediatrics, Elk Grove Village, IL, 1994.
Excellent reference book for all practices to have on hand; it covers symptoms, diagnosis, and management.

Woolf, AD: Poisoning in children and adolescents. Pediatrics in Review 14:411–422, 1993.
Comprehensive review of all aspects of childhood poisoning, including clinical and examination clues for specific classes of poisons. Bibliography is categorized by specific and common poisonings.

Chapter 24: Rashes

Frieden, IJ: Childhood exanthems. Current Opinion in Pediatrics 7:411–414, 1995.
Comprehensive review of childhood rashes with update on several new aspects, including the relationship between parvovirus B19 infection and papular-purpuric gloves and socks syndrome.

Resnick, SD: New aspects of exanthematous diseases of childhood. Dermatologic Clinics 15:257–266, 1997.
Excellent review of new exanthems and the importance of immunization for measles and varicella.

Singleton, JK: Pediatric dermatosis: Three common skin disruptions in infancy. Nurse Practitioner 22:32–33, 43–44, 1997.
The diagnostic and management considerations for seborrheic dermatitis, diaper rash, and atopic dermatitis are reviewed in detail.

Chapter 25: Sore Throat

Pichichero, ME: Sore throat after sore throat after sore throat. Are you asking the critical questions? Post-graduate Medicine 101:209–212, 1997.

The causes and management of recurrent group A streptococcal infections are reviewed with a discussion of the differential diagnosis of treatment failure.

Ruppert, SD: Differential diagnosis of common causes of pediatric pharyngitis. Nurse Practitioner 21: 38–42, 1996.

The common causes of sore throat are reviewed, including group A and nongroup A streptococci, viral pharyngitis, and infectious mononucleosis.

Wald, ER, et al: A streptococcal score card revisited. Pediatric Emergency Care 14:109–111, 1998.

This article presents the positive predictive value of a six-point clinical score card for diagnosing the likeli-hood that a throat culture will be positive for group A streptococci.

Chapter 26: Strains and Sprains

Hergenroeder, AC: Diagnosis and treatment of ankle sprains. A review. American Journal of Diseases of Children 144:809–814, 1990.

Clinicians should be more engaged in the management of musculoskeletal trauma in young athletes. This article, which reviews the basic principles of diagnosis and management, should help.

Innis, PC: Office evaluation and treatment of finger and hand injuries in children. Current Opinion in Pediatrics 7:83–87, 1995.

Pediatric finger and wrist injuries are common. Good outcome will depend upon appropriate diagnosis and management of sprains and fractures.

Wexler, RK: The injured ankle. American Family Physician 57:474–480, 1998.

Treatment options are reviewed, differentiating injuries that can be treated in office primary care versus those that are more serious and should be referred to an orthopedic specialist.

Chapter 27: Urinary Burning and Frequency

Hellerstein, S: Urinary tract infections: Old and new concepts. Pediatric Clinics of North America 42:1433–1457, 1995.

Recommendations for evaluation and treatment of pediatric UTI and a discussion of children who are at greatest risk for renal damage.

Hoberman, A, and Wald, ER: Urinary tract infections in young children: New light on old questions. Contemporary Pediatrics 14:140–156, 1997.

These authoritative authors present their views on the controversies of evaluation and management of UTI in infants and children, and the basis for decisions regarding testing as well as screening.

Robson, WL, and Leung, AK: Extraordinary urinary frequency syndrome (EUFS). Urology 42:321–324, 1993.

The authors report their experience with 31 children who were diagnosed with EUFS, with a focus on etiology.

Chapter 28: Vomiting

First, L: Nausea and vomiting. In Gellis, S, and Kagan, B (eds): Current Pediatric Therapy, ed 15. WB Saunders, Philadelphia, 1996, pp 266–268.

A complete review of mechanisms, causes, and management of vomiting in all age groups, including the use of drugs to control vomiting. The emphasis is on finding a cause before starting treatment.

Ramos, A, and Tuchman, D: Persistent vomiting. Pediatrics in Review 15:24–30, 1994.

Review article discussing mechanisms that control vomiting, age-related differences in etiology, and the appropriate use of antiemetics.

Winter, N: Vomiting in Ambulatory Pediatric Care. In Dershewitz, RA (ed): Ambulatory Pediatric Care, ed 3. Lippincott-Raven, Philadelphia 1999, pp 566–569.

Comprehensive discussion of clinical presentation, differential diagnosis, management, and indication for referral in children with vomiting.

Chapter 29: Wounds

Brokaw, A, and Ellwood, L: Planning for pediatric laceration repairs. Nurse Practitioner 21:42–49, 1996.
Article discusses repair techniques and how to manage the uncooperative child.

Sectish, TC: Use of sedation and local anesthesia to prepare children for procedures. American Family Physician 55:909–916, 1997.
Selective use of sedation and the need for newer topical agents for local anesthesia are discussed based on the child's age and degree of cooperation.

Shafi, S, and Gilbert, JC: Minor pediatric injuries. Pediatric Clinics of North America 45:831–851, 1998.
Good review of principles of wound care and appropriate closure of the wound to optimize healing.

SYMPTOMS IN ADULTS

Chapter 30: Abdominal Pain

Apstein, MD, and Carey, MC: Gallstones. In Branch, WT, Jr (ed): Office Practice of Medicine, ed 3. WB Saunders, Philadelphia, 1994, pp 277–295.
This chapter describes another common cause of abdominal pain in adults. It outlines the pathogenesis of gallstones, the symptoms of acute and chronic cholecystitis, and its medical and surgical management.

Bynum, TE, and Branch, WT: Dyspepsia and upper abdominal pain. In Branch, WT, Jr (ed): Office Practice of Medicine, ed 3. WB Saunders, Philadelphia, 1994, pp 255–276.
This chapter reviews the pathophysiology of these two very common causes of adult abdominal pain. It also provides algorithms to guide evaluation and treatment.

Silen, W: Abdominal pain. In Fauci, AS, et al (eds): Harrison's Principles of Internal Medicine, ed 14. McGraw-Hill, New York, 1998, pp 65–68.
This chapter is a concise overview of the many causes of abdominal pain, written by a master surgeon who brings years of experience to the challenge of correctly diagnosing this symptom.

Chapter 31: Allergic Reactions and Anaphylaxis

Bochner, BS, and Lichtenstein, LM: Anaphylaxis. N Engl J Med 324:1785–1790, 1991.
This is an excellent brief review of anaphylaxis, clinical presentation, causes, and treatment.

Kemp, SF, et al: Anaphylaxis: A review of 266 cases. Archives of Internal Medicine 155:1749–1754, 1995.
This paper is an excellent review of 266 individuals presenting as outpatients with a history of anaphylaxis. Details regarding clinical backgrounds, the frequency of recurrence, clinical presentations, and causes are well outlined. This summary provides an excellent clinical background on anaphylaxis.

Nicklas, RA, et al: The diagnosis and management of anaphylaxis. Journal of Allergy and Clinical Immunology 101(Suppl):S465–S528, 1998.
This supplement is a practice parameter publication. It includes invaluable outlines, including an algorithm for initial evaluation and treatment of anaphylaxis, definition of anaphylaxis, and advice regarding evaluation. Brief outlines and references are available for major causes of anaphylaxis, including medications, insect stings, foods, and others. This is an excellent starting point for anyone dealing with anaphylaxis.

Chapter 32: Back Pain

Bigos, SJ, et al: Acute Low Back Problems in Adults: Clinical Practice Guidelines No. 14. Agency for Healthcare Research and Quality, Rockville, MD. AHCPR Publication 95-0642, 1994. Available at http://www.ahrq.gov/clinic/cpgonline.htm. Accessed January 3, 2001.
A consensus statement by a panel of back pain experts assembled by the U.S. government.

Frymoyer, JW, et al: Back pain and sciatica. N Engl J Med 318:291–300, 1988.
An excellent general review of back pain.

National Guideline Clearinghouse Web site. Available at http://www.guidelines.gov. Accessed January 3, 2001.
A collection of evidence-based clinical practice guidelines, including those for acute low back pain, prepared by various groups.

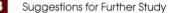

Chapter 33: Breast Pain in Nursing Mothers

Huggins K: The Nursing Mother's Companion, ed 3. Harvard Community Press, Cambridge, MA, 1995.
A chronological guide to the breastfeeding process in the developing infant. Topics are a bit more difficult to find, but this is a complete guide for patients.

La Leche League International: The Womanly Art of Breastfeeding. Penguin Group, New York, 1997. Chapter 7, "Common Concerns."
The definitive guide for the breastfeeding mother, this reference should be on the shelf of anyone who cares for postpartum women. Chapter 7 covers breast pumps, sore nipples, breast infections, etc.

Moody, J, et al: Breastfeeding Your Baby. Fisher Books, Tucson, AZ, 1997. Chapter 8, "Breast Troubles." Chapter 9, "Nursing Problems."
Billed as "advice from over 200 women," this book serves as a practical guide with many pictures and diagrams.

Spock B, and Rothenberg, MB: Dr. Spock's Baby and Child Care, ed 7. Simon & Schuster, New York, 1998.
The classic home reference, Dr. Spock's book still has concise, practical information, listed by topic for easy reference. There is an excellent section on breastfeeding.

Chapter 34: Burns

Sabiston, D: Textbook of Surgery. The Biological Basis of Modern Surgical Practice. WB Saunders, Philadelphia, 1997, pp 221–223.
A comprehensive surgical text. Has great up-to-date information on all varieties of surgical problems. Its length looks overwhelming, but it is very readable and understandable to many levels of clinicians.

Saunders, CE, and Ho, MT: Current Emergency Diagnosis & Treatment, ed 4. Appleton & Lange, East Norwalk, CT, 1992, pp 691–702.
Very thorough text for all types of emergencies from the simple to the complex. Gives good information on diagnosis and treatment. Well organized and easy to read.

Trott, AT: Wounds and Lacerations: Emergency Care and Closure, ed 2. Mosby–Year Book, St. Louis, 1997, pp 302–309, 358–359.
Great text to keep in the office. Very practically oriented to caring for wounds of many types. Also has very good, clear instructions on caring for these wounds. Easy to read and understand.

Chapter 35: Chest Pain

Braunwald, E: Examination of the patient. The history. In Braunwald, E (ed): Heart Disease: A Textbook of Cardiovascular Medicine, ed 5. WB Saunders, Philadelphia, 1997, pp 3–7.
Excellent description of chest pain caused by myocardial infarction and coronary insufficiency, in one of the best books on cardiovascular disorders. This chapter has a very nice table of associated symptoms and tricks for differentiating MI from noncardiac pain.

Christie, LG, and Conti, CR: Systematic approach to evaluation of angina-like chest pain. American Heart Journal 102:897, 1981.
Gives a good flavor of angina with graphic description, which has not changed in the past 20 years.

Constant, J: The clinical diagnosis of nonanginal chest pain. Clinical Cardiology 6:11, 1983.
A cogent discussion of causes for chest pain other than angina or MI. A resource used by all the current textbooks.

O'Rourke, RA, et al: The history, physical, and cardiac auscultation. In Alexander, RW, et al (eds): The Heart, ed 9. McGraw-Hill, New York, 1998, pp 231–236.
A classic about cardiovascular disorders from the old school of teachers who could make the diagnosis from signs and symptoms without the fancy tests available now.

Chapter 36: Colds and Flu

DuBuske, LM, and Sheffer, AL: Allergic rhinitis and other diseases of the nose. In Branch, WT (ed): Office Practice of Medicine, ed 3. WB Saunders, Philadelphia, 1994, pp 176–185.
A discussion of allergic nasal symptoms.

Kirkpatrick, GL: Viral infections of the respiratory tract. In Taylor, RB (ed): Family Medicine Principles and Practice, ed 5. Springer-Verlag, New York, 1997, pp 328–336.

A general introduction to common colds, bronchitis, and flu.

Williams, JW, and Simel, DL: Sinusitis. In Dornbrand, L, et al (eds): Manual of Clinical Problems in Adult Ambulatory Care, ed 3. Lippincott-Raven, Philadelphia, 1997, pp 72–76.

A specific discussion of the cause and treatment of sinus infections.

Chapter 37: Constipation

Abyad, A, and Mourad, F: Constipation: Common-sense care of the older patient. Geriatrics 51(12):28–36, 1996.

Although focused on the elderly, this article is relevant to any adult patient. It contains excellent descriptions of medications commonly used for constipation, their doses and side effects. The article includes a table with a sensible stepwise approach to management.

Koch, TR: Constipation. In Haubrich, WS, et al (eds): Bockus Gastroenterology, ed 5. WB Saunders, Philadelphia, 1995, pp 102–112.

This chapter discusses the physiologic causes of constipation and gives recommendations for medical evaluation and management.

Chapter 38: Cough

Mello, CJ, et al: Predictive value of the character, timing, and complications of chronic cough in diagnosing its cause. Archives of Internal Medicine 156:997–1003, 1996.

This article and the one following, by Pratter et al., are both excellent and comprehensive reviews of evaluating the causes of chronic cough.

Pratter, MR, et al: An algorithmic approach to chronic cough. Annals of Internal Medicine 119:977–983, 1993.

Chapter 39: Diarrhea

Surawicz, CM: Diarrhea. In Dale, DC, and Federman, DD (eds): Scientific American Medicine, Vol. 1, Tab 4, Section III, Diarrhea. Scientific American, New York, 1998, pp 1–10.

This is a well-written, thorough article that details the pathophysiology and recommended treatments of all causes of diarrhea. It is organized in order of prevalance, discussing the common causes first.

Web sites with regularly updated information about acute and chronic diarrhea and on foodborne pathogens include the Centers for Disease Control and Prevention (http://www.cdc.gov), the Food and Drug Administration (http://www.fda.gov), the American Gastroenterological Association (http://www.gastro.org), and the American College of Gastroenterology (http://acg.org).

These sites are particularly useful if one is interested in learning about epidemics of diarrhea in different areas of the country and the world. Patients sometimes call, concerned about epidemics about which they have heard via the news media.

Chapter 40: Ear Pain

Fry, TL: Earwax. In Dornbrand, et al (eds): Manual of Clinical Problems in Adult Ambulatory Care, ed 3. Lippincott-Raven, Philadelphia, 1997, pp 62–64.

A discussion of how to manage ear wax buildup.

Gulya, AJ: Approach to the patient with otitis. In Goroll, AH, et al (eds): Primary Care Medicine: Office Evaluation and Management of the Adult Patient, ed 3. JB Lippincott, Philadelphia, 1995, pp 1002–1004.

A good short summary of management of otitis media and externa in adults.

La Rosa, S: Primary care management of otitis externa. Nurse Practitioner 23:125–128, 131–133, 1998.

The causes, complications, and treatment of swimmer's ear.

Chapter 41: Eye Pain and Foreign Bodies

Bradford, CA: Basic Ophthalmology for Medical Students and Primary Care Residents. American Academy of Ophthalmology, San Francisco, 1999.

> *This is one of the best short textbooks written for non-ophthalmologists. It is a great text for physicians in training and an excellent reference for primary care physicians, nurse practitioners, and physician assistants.*

Trobe, JD: The Physician's Guide to Eye Care: How to Diagnose, How to Treat, When to Refer. American Academy of Ophthalmology, San Francisco, 1993.

> *This concise but comprehensive manual was written in collaboration with primary care physicians. The book is organized around common clinical challenges. If you are planning to get one book to help you deal with "front-line" eye problems, this is the one to get. Excellent color photos, illustrations, tables, and step-by-step instructions enhance the text.*

Chapter 42: Fainting

Kapoor, WN: Evaluation and management of patients with syncope. JAMA 268:2553–2560, 1992.

> *A review by one of the leading scholars of syncope, with an emphasis on the care of patients with more severe and difficult-to-manage syncope.*

Lipsitz, L: Orthostatic hypotension in the elderly. N Engl J Med 321:952–956, 1989.

> *The elderly are especially prone to syncope from both harmless and dangerous causes.*

Chapter 43: Fever

Breeling, J, and Weinstein, L: Fever of unknown origin. In Branch, WT (ed): Office Practice of Medicine, ed 3. WB Saunders, Philadelphia, 1994, p 845.

> *This contains a complete discussion of fever of unknown origin as it presents in the outpatient setting.*

Gelfund, J, et al: Fever. In Harrison, TR (ed-): Harrison's Principles of Internal Medicine, ed 13. McGraw-Hill, New York, 1994, pp 81–90.

> *All the references listed here offer a good general discussion of fever and its causes. Harrison's textbook provides a more in-depth discussion of fever pathophysiology.*

Lipsky, B: Fever. In Film, S, and McGee, S (eds): Outpatient Medicine. WB Saunders, Philadelphia, 1992, p 60.

> *A slightly more basic and brief overview of fever in outpatients.*

Chapter 44: Frostbite

Sabiston, D: Textbook of Surgery. The Biological Basis of Modern Surgical Practice. WB Saunders, Philadelphia, 1997, pp 246–250.

> *A comprehensive surgical text. Has great up-to-date information on all varieties of surgical problems, including frostbite. Its length looks overwhelming, but it is very readable and understandable to many levels of clinicians.*

Saunders, CE, and Ho, MT: Current Emergency Diagnosis & Treatment, ed 4. Appleton & Lange, East Norwalk, CT, 1992, pp 705–709.

> *Very thorough text for all types of emergencies from the simple to the complex. Gives good information on diagnosis and treatment of all types of wounds, including frostbite. Well organized and easy to read.*

Chapter 45: Headache

Lance, JW: Mechanism and Management of Headache, ed 5. Butterworth, London, 1993.

> *This is the gold standard in the diagnosis and treatment of headache disorders.*

Silverstein, SD: Evaluation and emergency treatment of headache. Headache 32:396–407, 1992.

> *This is an excellent article on the evaluation and treatment of acute headache syndromes.*

Chapter 46: Head Injury

Hafen, BQ: Injuries. In First Aid for Health Emergencies, ed 3. West Publishing, St. Paul, MN, 1985, pp 139–181.
  Detailed description of head injuries and head wounds with first aid and follow-up treatment. Chapter includes general wounds, foreign bodies, and other traumatic injuries.

Head Injuries. In Athletic Training and Sports Medicine, ed 2. American Academy of Orthopaedic Surgeons, Park Ridge, IL, 1991, pp 496–505.
  This chapter focuses on common head injuries. It includes a discussion on assessing head injuries.

Chapter 47: Menstrual Cycle Problems: Amenorrhea and Oligomenorrhea

Boston Women's Health Book Collective: Our Bodies, Ourselves for the New Century. Simon & Schuster, New York, 1998. Chapter 12, "Understanding Our Bodies: Sexual Anatomy, Reproduction and the Menstrual Cycle."
  The classic self-help text. Chapter 12 is a good overview of normal reproduction written for a lay audience.

Carlson, K, et al: Harvard Guide to Women's Health. Harvard University Press, Cambridge, MA, 1996.
  A complete guide to women's health issues, this book contains a brief section on amenorrhea.

Slupik, R (ed): American Medical Association Complete Guide to Women's Health. Random House, New York, 1996. Chapter 7, "The Reproductive System and Menstrual Cycle."
  An excellent lay reference with clear pictures, diagrams, and decision trees, with advice on home care and when to see a physician.

Speroff, L, et al: Clinical Gynecologic Endocrinology and Infertility, ed 4. Williams & Wilkins, Baltimore, 1989. Chapter 5, "Amenorrhea," pp 165–212.
  An excellent, though scholarly, overview of various causes of amenorrhea and their workup.

Chapter 48: Menstrual Pain

Boston Women's Health Book Collective: Our Bodies, Ourselves. Simon & Schuster, New York, 1998.
  This is an excellent general resource covering all aspects of women's health and well-being in a style that patients can easily comprehend.

Carlson, K, et al: Harvard Guide to Women's Health. Harvard University Press, Cambridge, MA, 1996.
  A somewhat more technical reference that does a good job of explaining the medical aspects of women's health conditions.

Northrup, C: Women's Bodies, Women's Wisdom. Bantam Books, New York, 1998.
  A wonderful general reference that also includes holistic aproaches to women's health issues.

Chapter 49: Neck Pain

Afeiche, NE: Neck pain. In Barker, LR, et al (eds): Ambulatory Medicine. Williams & Wilkins, Baltimore, 1991, pp 806–814.
  An excellent source of outpatient management, which includes several useful patient exercises.

Nakano, KK: Neck pain. In Kelley, WM, et al (eds): Textbook of Rheumatology. WB Saunders, Philadelphia, 1989, pp 471–491.
  A detailed review of anatomy, physiology, and treatment, with excellent figures and tables.

Chapter 50: Nosebleed

Wegmaller, E: Emergencies of the ear, facial structure, and upper airway. In Wilkins, E (ed): MGH Textbook of Emergency Medicine, ed 2. Williams & Wilkins, Baltimore, 1983.

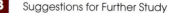
Wilson, W: Approach to epistaxis. In Goroll, A, et al (eds): Primary Care Medicine: Office Evaluation and Management of the Adult Patient, ed 3. JB Lippincott, Philadelphia, 1995.

Chapter 51: Rashes and Infestations

Fitzpatrick, TB, et al: Color Atlas and Synopsis of Clinical Dermatology: Common and Serious Diseases, ed 3. McGraw-Hill, New York, 1997, pp 836–849.
   This book summarizes presenting symptoms and treatment for head lice, crab lice, and scabies, with pictures of the typical physical findings.

Fitzpatrick, TB, and Johnson, RA: Emergency management of patients with rash and fever. In Wilkins, E (ed): MGH Textbook of Emergency Medicine, ed 2. Williams & Wilkins, Baltimore, 1983.

Goldsmith, LA, et al: Adult and Pediatric Dermatology: A Color Guide to Diagnosis and Treatment. FA Davis, Philadelphia, 1997.
   Basic information on a wide range of skin lesions, arranged by appearance so they can be located without knowing the diagnosis in advance.

http://www.headlice.org
   This well-designed Website is the home page of the National Pediculosis Association, a nonprofit health education agency. The association collects and disseminates information about effectiveness and safety of treatments and maintains a registry for reporting outbreaks, treatment failures, and adverse reactions to treatment. It has excellent practical suggestions for families dealing with resistant lice infestations and for mechanical removal of lice and nits. Some of their educational information is available in Spanish. The association also can be contacted at National Pediculosis Association, Inc., P.O. Box 610189, Newton, MA 02161, or 781-449-NITS.

Reeves, JRT, and Maibach, HI: Clinical Dermatology Illustrated: A Regional Approach, ed 3. FA Davis, Philadelphia, 1998.
   Skin conditions grouped by location on the body; includes patient guides for common disorders.

Chapter 52: Shortness of Breath

Cohn, JN: The management of congestive heart failure. N Engl J Med 335:490–498, 1996.

Ferguson, GT, and Cherniack, RM: Management of chronic obstructive pulmonary disease. N Engl J Med 328:1017–1022, 1993.

McFadden, ER, Jr, and Gilbert, IA: Asthma. N Engl J Med 327:1928–1936, 1992.
   These three articles review the pathophysiology and treatment of the three main causes of shortness of breath.

Chapter 53: Sore Throat

Centor, RM: Sore throat. In Dornbrand, L, et al (eds): Manual of Clinical Problems in Adult Ambulatory Care, ed 3. Lippincott-Raven, Philadelphia, 1997, pp 76–82.
   A practical approach to diagnosing and treating sore throats.

Komaroff, AL, et al: The prediction of streptococcal pharyngitis in adults. Journal of General Internal Medicine 1:1–7, 1986.
   Decision guidelines as to when a culture is and is not useful in diagnosing strep throat in adults.

Schwartz, B, and O'Brien, KL: Streptococcal infections. In Kelly, WN (ed): Textbook of Internal Medicine, ed, 3. Lippincott-Raven, Philadelphia, 1997, pp 1614–1616.
   The cause, consequences, and treatment of strep throat.

Chapter 54: Strains and Sprains

Fredericson, M: Common injuries in runners. Diagnosis, rehabilitation and prevention. Sports Medicine 21(1):49–72, 1996.
   Runners get frequent lower extremity injuries, and this review is a useful guide to recognition and treatment of these commonly seen problems.

Jardon, OM, and Matthews, MS: Orthopedics. In Rakel, RE (ed): Textbook of Family Practice, ed 5. WB Saunders, Philadelphia, 1995, pp 917–968.

A discussion of the different injury syndromes encountered in primary care.

Lillegard, WA, et al: Common upper extremity injuries. Archives of Family Medicine 5:159–168 1996.

A review of how to treat minor upper extremity injuries and how to recognize the more serious ones that require referral to a specialist.

Tuggy, ML, and Breuner, CC: Athletic injuries. In Taylor, RB (ed): Family Medicine Principles and Practice, ed 5. Springer-Verlag, New York, 1997, pp 453–464.

A discussion of the most common athletic injuries.

Chapter 55: Sunburn

Sabiston, D: Textbook of Surgery. The Biological Basis of Modern Surgical Practice. WB Saunders, Philadelphia, 1997, pp 245–246.

A comprehensive surgical text. Has great up-to-date information on all varieties of surgical problems. Its length looks overwhelming, but it is very readable and understandable to many levels of clinicians.

Saunders, CE, and Ho, MT: Current Emergency Diagnosis & Treatment, ed 4. Appleton & Lange, East Norwalk, CT, 1992, p 700.

Very thorough text for all types of emergencies from the simple to the complex. Gives good information on diagnosis and treatment. Well organized and easy to read.

Trott, AT: Wounds and Lacerations: Emergency Care and Closure, ed 2. Mosby–Year Book, St. Louis, 1997, pp 302–309.

Great text to keep in the office. Very practically oriented to caring for wounds of many types. Also has very good, clear instructions on caring for these wounds. Easy to read and understand.

Chapter 56: Urinary Tract Infections

Hooton, TM, et al: A prospective study of risk factors for symptomatic urinary tract infection in young women. N Engl J Med 335:468, 1996.

This study identifies recent intercourse, use of diaphragm and spermicide, and history of recurrent urinary tract infections as risk factors for symptomatic urinary tract infections in sexually active young women.

Stamm, WE, and Hooton, TM: Management of urinary tract infections in adults. N Engl J Med 329:1328–1334, 1993.

This is an excellent review of urinary tract infections in adults, emphasizing cost-effective management strategies.

Chapter 57: Vaginal Bleeding

Bayer, SR, and DeCherney, AH: Clinical manifestations and treatment of dysfunctional uterine bleeding. JAMA 269:1823–1828, 1993.

A concise overview of the presentation and treatment of dysfunctional uterine bleeding, the most common cause of vaginal bleeding in women of reproductive age.

Jennings, JC: Abnormal uterine bleeding. Medical Clinics of North America 79(6):1357–1376, 1995.

A complete review of causes, diagnostic evaluation, and management of abnormal uterine bleeding. The discussion covers patients ranging in age from adolescence through the menopause.

Chapter 58: Vaginal Discharge

Carr, PL, et al: Evaluation and management of vaginitis. Journal of General Internal Medicine 13:335–346, 1998.

Recent review of diagnosis and treatment of vaginitis.

Kent, HL: Epidemiology of vaginitis. American Journal of Obstetrics and Gynecology 165:1168–1176, 1991.

An excellent overview of vaginal infections in women and the epidemiologic associations of the various causes.

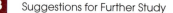

Chapter 59: Visual Disturbance

Berson, FG: Basic Ophthalmology for Medical Students and Primary Care Residents. American Academy of Ophthalmology, San Francisco, 1993.
> *This is one of the best short textbooks written for nonophthalmologists. It is a great text for physicians in training and an excellent reference for primary care physicians, nurse practitioners, and physician assistants.*

Sacks, O: Migraine. University of California Press, Berkeley, CA, 1992.
> *A comprehensive treatment of migraine headaches by the well-known neurologist-author. It should be of interest both to those who suffer from migraine and those who treat it.*

Trobe, JD: The Physician's Guide to Eye Care: How to Diagnose, How to Treat, When to Refer. American Academy of Ophthalmology, San Francisco, 1993.
> *This concise but comprehensive manual was written in collaboration with primary care physicians. The book is organized around common clinical challenges. If you are planning to get one book to help you deal with "front-line" eye problems, this is the one to get. Excellent color photos, illustrations, tables, and step-by-step instructions enhance the text.*

Chapter 60: Vomiting and Nausea

Hanson, JS, and McCallum, RW: The diagnosis and managment of nausea and vomiting: A review. American Journal of Gastroenterology 80:210, 1985.
> *Good review of the physiological basis for vomiting and its diagnosis and management.*

Levine, JS: Decision Making in Gastroenterology, ed 2. CV Mosby, St. Louis, 1992, pp 72–74.
> *Short algorithms for clinicians.*

Sleisenger, MH, and Fordtran, JS: Gastrointestinal and Liver Disease. Pathophysiology, Diagnosis, and Management, ed 6. WB Saunders, Philadelphia, 1998, pp 117–126.
> *Written for internists and subspecialists. Markedly detailed and complete information.*

Yamada, T: Approach to the patient with nausea and vomiting. In Yamada, T. (ed): Textbook of Gastroenterology, ed 2, Vol. I. JB Lippincott, Philadelphia, 1995, pp 731–743.
> *Another thorough physiologic review.*

Chapter 61: Wheezing

McFadden, ER, Jr, and Gilbert, IA: Asthma. N Engl J Med 327:1928–1936, 1992.
> *Excellent general review.*

McFadden, ER, Jr, and Gilbert, IA: Exercise-induced asthma. N Engl J Med 330:1362–1366, 1994.
> *A review of the physiology and treatment of this disorder.*

Spitzer, WO, et al: The use of β-agonists and the risk of death and near death from asthma. N Engl J Med 326:501–506, 1992.
> *Excessive use of inhaled bronchodilators can place patients at high risk of sudden cardiac death.*

Chapter 62: Wounds

American Academy of Orthopaedic Surgeons (Briese, GL, ed.): First Responder. Jones and Bartlett Publishers, Sudbury, MA, 1997, pp 296–307.
> *Thorough, concise description of wounds, wound care, and treatment principles including specific wound treatment. Overall, a good reference for first aid and triage. Includes self-tests.*

Cosgriff, JH, Jr, and Anderson, D: Management of wounds and bites. In Cosgriff, JH, and Anderson, D (eds): The Practice of Emergency Nursing. JB Lippincott, Philadelphia, 1975, pp 121–139.
> *A good review with discussion of wound assessment, management, and healing physiology. Includes prophylaxis guidelines.*

Schafermeyer, RW: Minor trauma. In Harwood-Nuss, A, et al: (eds): The Clinical Practice of Emergency Medicine. JB Lippincott, Philadelphia, 1991, pp 841–846.
Discussion of epidemiology, evaluation, management, and pitfalls. Includes associated injuries and animal bites.

Sheehy, SB: Wound management. In Manual of Emergency Care: Principles and Practice, ed 3. CV Mosby, St. Paul, MN, 1990, pp 350–365.
Thorough chapter on wound types, therapeutic intervention, antiseptic solutions, and wound healing.

Index

Page numbers followed by an "f" indicate a figure. Page numbers followed by a "t" indicate a table.